Notice

The content of this book has been written for informational and discussion purposes only. Although the reader may find the ideas, concepts, suggestions, and recommendations useful, they are provided on the understanding that neither the author nor the publisher is qualified or engaged to provide specific medical, dietary, nutrition, or health advice to the reader. Each person has unique medical, dietary, nutrition, and health requirements which each reader should discuss with his or her doctor, dietician, nutritionist, or healthcare professional.

No part of this book may be copied, reproduced, distributed, or transmitted by any means, including digital, mechanical, photocopying, recording, or otherwise, without the advance written permission of the author.

ISBN: 1499246803
ISBN-13: 9781499246803

Library of Congress Control Number: 2014907978
CreateSpace Independent Publishing Platform
North Charleston, South Carolina

STOP EATING THE ANIMALS

An Appeal on Behalf of The Voiceless to Adopt a Meat-Free Foodstyle

JERRY H. PARISELLA

DEDICATION

This book is dedicated to my wife, Anna, who has done the heavy lifting in applying her culinary skills to create so many flavorful, nutritious meat-free dishes. Eating in our home is never a bore but an event to eagerly anticipate. Most appreciated is the TLC that she puts into every dish, which is true nourishment for the soul.

Credit is due to the "Ambassadors of the Animal Kingdom," who taught me to pay attention to animals in ways that I hadn't considered before: Buba, our determined Dachshund who, even in her old age with her faculties failing, always kept herself moving, teaching us a lesson to remain active in order to sustain our own health; Arkasha, her endearing son who had an irresistible way of grabbing my attention that evolved into a level of mutual understanding that I never would have imagined possible between a human and an animal; and Mishka, our young, adopted male Dachshund who amazes my wife and me with his ability to "train" us to accommodate his preferences and to evoke affectionate responses that surprise even us.

Not unlike the pets who often provide the only substantive interaction with animals that most humans experience, each of our canine family members has served as an effective Ambassador of the Animal Kingdom, teaching us how very much they and every animal love life and deserve to live it fully and without infliction of suffering by humans.

My thanks to the scientists, doctors, philosophers, animal welfare advocates, journalists, photographers, undercover investigators, animal sanctuary operators, vegetarians, and vegans who have each contributed to a growing awareness of the deleterious effects of human consumption of animal flesh, of the sentience of our fellow creatures, of the systematic horrors inflicted by factory farming, and of how our flawed thinking desperately needs to undergo a paradigm shift.

As more people advocate for our voiceless fellow creatures, for human health, and for our shared environment, it is my hope that we will reach a tipping point for transcultural adoption of a meat-free foodstyle, the most healthy, ethical, and compassionate way to nourish ourselves.

May all humans become more humane.

Ad Maiorem Dei Gloriam

CONTENTS

INTRODUCTION

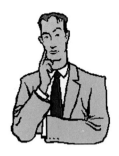

What's not to like about a filet mignon with bernaise sauce, foie gras with a glass of sauterne, or al dente spaghetti with veal meatballs? What's more mouth watering than a juicy cheeseburger on a toasted bun, apple-stuffed grilled sausages, or barbecued pulled pork? Who doesn't have fond memories of digging into tender roast turkey at Thanksgiving, slicing into a succulent baked ham at Easter, or pigging out on pepperoni pizza and cold beers with your friends?

Meat has been satiating our taste buds our entire lives, has been integrated into our holiday celebrations for generations, and has the power to make us salivate like Pavlovian dogs. Let's face it: meat tastes good, is full of nutrients, and has been an enjoyable part of our culture and social life.

Our lust for animal flesh is also compromising our health. It's inducing chronic inflammation in our cells, clogging our arteries, slowing our digestion, contributing to colon cancer, and making us fat.

Factory farms are supplying us with all that meat that causes the needless suffering of millions of animals who are forced to live miserable lives where they are unable to engage in natural animal behaviors and endure painful mutilations before facing horrific deaths and disassembly of their bodies.

Our insatiable demand for the flesh of animals and its ready supply from industrial-scale factory farms also undermines efforts to feed the world's starving and malnourished humans by inefficiently using limited agricultural land to raise animals for slaughter, land that could otherwise be more efficiently used to grow nutritious plants and grains for wider human consumption. This is not inconsequential in a world where 870 million of our fellow human beings are hungry, two billion are nutritionally deficient, and twenty million die each year from starvation or diseases related to malnutrition.

Perhaps the two most pernicious prices that we all pay for remaining in this rarely questioned unholy alliance of animal eaters and animal slaughterers are the deadening of our hearts to the legitimate needs of others and habituating our minds to ignore the real costs of our self-indulgence.

To eat animal flesh is to encourage the killing of innocent animals. We may not wish ill for any animal and may, indeed, keep some animals as beloved pets. But the unavoidable calculus in an economy built on supply and demand is that the more steaks we buy at the supermarket, the more veal dishes we order at the restaurant, and the more burgers we throw on the grill, the more animals that will suffer and be slaughtered for their flesh. That is the truth.

To eat animals is more than just a simple dietary choice. It is a moral decision with existential consequences. It is difficult to initially appreciate this fact, since most factory farming is hidden from consumers' view, hindering our ability to make fully informed moral decisions about our dietary choices.

The purpose of this book, then, is to lay out a comprehensive case on behalf of the animals who, if we humans could understand their languages, would ask us to stop eating them.

As you think about the unintended, but no less real, consequences of which foods you choose to put into your mouth, may your heart be moved and your mind opened.

1
THE HEALTH EFFECTS OF EATING THE ANIMALS

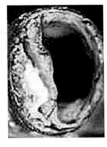

Clogged Artery

When we eat meat, we are eating the skeletal muscle and associated fat and other tissues of animals. Some people also eat offal, the internal organs and entrails (intestines) of animals. What visibly distinguishes red meat from white meat is the concentration of myoglobin, an iron and oxygen binding protein found in muscle tissue. When myoglobin is exposed to oxygen, reddish oxymyoglobin develops, making the meat appear red. Red meat – the muscles of adult mammals like cows, sheep, goats, and horses - contains more narrow muscle fibers that perform longer without rest, while white meat – such as the breast muscles of chickens and turkeys - contains more broad muscle fibers that function better in short bursts.

Meat is very high in fat, especially saturated fat, which is linked to fat deposits in our arteries, increased blood pressure, and artery damage. Since animal fat is the most calorie-dense nutrient, meat contains the fat most responsible for dangerous weight gain. Moreover, meat is very high in cholesterol. Our bodies produce enough cholesterol for human health. Eating animals' cholesterol increases the cholesterol load on our bodies and makes it more difficult to regulate without an assist from pharmaceutical intervention, such as the increasingly prescribed and profitable statin drugs.

Meat takes a long time to pass through our intestines, where it putrefies, producing toxins and amines that accumulate in the liver, kidneys, and large intestines and causes degeneration of the lining of the small intestine. Moreover, researchers have discovered that when meat is exposed to high temperatures during cooking, it produces carcinogenic compounds. These factors create the perfect storm to increase one's risk for developing colon or other cancers.

Since certain animal proteins are closely related to human proteins, our bodies respond to some as foreign and try to destroy them. When this happens repeatedly through regular meat consumption, some researchers believe the body may begin to turn on itself through autoimmune processes that may lead to the development of arthritis, lupus, and multiple sclerosis.

Unless the animals slaughtered were raised on organic farms, the animals were most likely injected with hormones to accelerate their growth and size. The faster animals grow and the more meat on their bodies, the more money that can be made. Unfortunately, most of the hormones injected are growth hormones that we take into our bodies when we eat an animal's flesh. Evidence is growing that this disrupts our own hormonal balances and may account for the increasingly early onset of puberty in our children.

In addition to hormones, most animals are also given antibiotics, which some believe may be contributing to the widely reported phenomenon of growing antibacterial resistance, whereby the antibiotics that we humans occasionally need are no longer as effective as they once were because bacteria have gotten so much exposure to them in small doses that the bacteria mutate against them.

Some health professionals believe that years of eating hard-to-digest, putrefying meat that moves very slowly through our stomach and intestines contributes to constipation, irritable bowel syndrome, and hemorrhoids.

Animals living in confined spaces, unable to perform the natural functions of their species, experience elevated, unrelenting stress that compromises their health and literally drives some animals mad. As fellow sentient beings, animals also sense danger and react accordingly.

This is no less true for factory farm animals who are led in lines to slaughter, seeing and hearing the suffering and deaths of their peers moments before their own premature deaths. This spike in stress hormones released into the animals' bodies escalates a series of biochemical reactions that become part of the animal flesh humans ultimately consume. In 2011, The Atlantic reported that The Journal of Animal Science and researchers at the University of Milan's Faculty of Veterinary Medicine confirmed that the fear which animals experience during slaughter significantly raises meat's levels of stress hormones – adrenaline, cortisol, and other steroids.

If you do the research, you will be amazed at the information coming in from the scientific community, particularly during the last two decades. In short, we now have enough data to know that eating animal flesh is harmful to us. Sure, we ingest some useful nutrients, including protein, iron, and vitamin B-12. But you may be surprised to know that we can get all the nutrients that we need from nonanimal sources. Much to the disbelief of many told otherwise, humans don't need to eat meat.

Science tells us that our entire lives—from fetus to infancy to adolescence to adulthood and through old age—can be lived healthily without consumption of animal flesh and body parts. We don't need to eat the animals.

The Academy of Nutrition and Dietetics, the world's largest organization of food and nutrition professionals, established in 1917 as the American Dietetic Association, issued the following position statement in 2009. It provides scientific reassurance that our nutritional needs can be completely met without resort to eating animal flesh.

Academy of Nutrition and Dietetics Position Statement

Vegetarian Diets

Volume 109, Issue 7, Pages 1266-1282 (July 2009)

Abstract

It is the position of the American Dietetic Association that appropriately planned vegetarian diets, including total vegetarian or vegan diets, are healthful, nutritionally adequate, and may provide health benefits in the prevention and treatment of certain diseases. Well-planned vegetarian diets are appropriate for individuals during all stages of the life cycle, including pregnancy, lactation, infancy, childhood, and adolescence, and for athletes. A vegetarian diet is defined as one that does not include meat (including fowl) or seafood, or products containing those foods. This article reviews the current data related to key nutrients for vegetarians including protein, n-3 fatty acids, iron, zinc, iodine, calcium, and vitamins D and B-12. A vegetarian diet can meet current recommendations for all of these nutrients. In some cases, supplements or fortified foods can provide useful amounts of important nutrients. An evidence-based review showed that vegetarian diets can be nutritionally adequate in pregnancy and result in positive maternal and infant health outcomes. The results of an evidence-based review showed that a vegetarian diet is associated with a lower risk of death from ischemic heart disease. Vegetarians also appear to have lower low-density lipoprotein cholesterol levels, lower blood pressure, and lower rates of hypertension and type

2 diabetes than nonvegetarians. Furthermore, vegetarians tend to have a lower body mass index and lower overall cancer rates. Features of a vegetarian diet that may reduce risk of chronic disease include lower intakes of saturated fat and cholesterol and higher intakes of fruits, vegetables, whole grains, nuts, soy products, fiber, and phytochemicals. The variability of dietary practices among vegetarians makes individual assessment of dietary adequacy essential. In addition to assessing dietary adequacy, food and nutrition professionals can also play key roles in educating vegetarians about sources of specific nutrients, food purchase and preparation, and dietary modifications to meet their needs.

© Academy of Nutrition and Dietetics

2
THE ANIMALS WE EAT

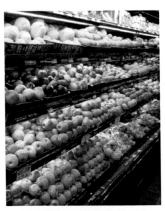

If you stroll through the typical grocery store, you'll see a wide variety of products in refrigerated cases, nicely displayed to pique our interest: sweet strawberries in clear plastic cases; beautiful portabella mushrooms stacked high for the picking; red, marbled steaks snugly packed in cellophane; strips of bacon nestled in vacuum-sealed pouches. The breadth of edible offerings seemingly has no limits, nor does the level of consumption convenience.

We can now purchase salads precut and premixed in ready-to-use plastic bags. We can have the deli worker slice a whole host of different beef, pork, fowl, or exotic luncheon meats for immediate layering

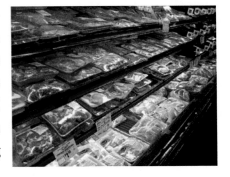

on our favorite sandwich rolls. We can skip purchasing, washing, and slicing individual fruits and simply opt for a premade fruit salad within its own disposable bowl. We can choose from among an array of meat sausages stuffed with all variety of fruits and herbs. We can even ask the butcher to save us the effort by slicing off excess fat from the steak that we'll take home to grill that evening.

While all of this packaging and convenience undoubtedly makes our lives easier, it also has the effect of impeding consumers from developing a full appreciation for the sources of their food. Although fruits and vegetables may be similarly displayed as cuts of meat, they come from very different sources. But you wouldn't know it from the way that they're presented to us at the store in a visual—and implied moral—equivalence between a vegetable and an animal.

We know that vegetables, fruits, legumes, nuts, and seeds are grown in or on the earth, are harvested with minimal subsequent effort required for their consumption, and never involve the infliction of pain or suffering. Indeed, except for accommodating shipping and distribution time, plants and grains are allowed to live out their natural lives until they are ripe for harvesting.

The meat products that we have politely renamed "steak," "sirloin," and "sausage" are actually body parts taken from sentient beings whose lives were lived in miserable confinement before being prematurely and horrifically ended on a factory production line of bloodletting and bodily disassembly too obscene to allow our children to see.

Why are we thrilled to show children how vegetables are grown on a farm or bring them to an orchard to pick fruits from trees, yet shield them from seeing a slaughterhouse and the carnage going on inside? Doesn't that speak volumes? It's hard not to imagine that if our children saw animals unnaturally confined and unceremoniously killed—their blood spilled, their bodies torn apart, and their flesh packaged for our tables—they would be asking their parents uncomfortable questions that we adults are often unwilling to ask ourselves.

Make no mistake about it, notwithstanding the clever names and pretty packaging, when we eat meat, we are eating the decaying flesh and body parts of animal corpses. It's not very appetizing when you think about what you are actually eating.

Just how obscene is the process of killing and disassembling innocent, living, breathing, playing, feeling animals into hunks of muscle, fat, and bone for us to

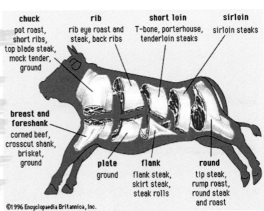

| chuck | rib | short loin | sirloin |
| pot roast, short ribs, top blade steak, mock tender, ground | rib eye roast and steak, back ribs | T-bone, porterhouse, tenderloin steaks | sirloin steaks |

breast and foreshank
corned beef, crosscut shank, brisket, ground

| plate | flank | round |
| ground | flank steak, skirt steak, steak rolls | tip steak, rump roast, round steak and roast |

©1996 Encyclopaedia Britannica, Inc.

eat? I invite adults to look at the investigations that such courageous nonprofits as Mercy For Animals (MFA), People for the Ethical Treatment of Animals (PETA), and the American Society for the Prevention of Cruelty to Animals (ASPCA), to name but a few, have conducted of factory farms.

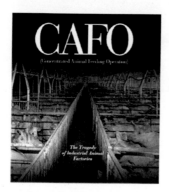

Or open the impressive tome edited by Daniel Imhoff, *CAFO: The Tragedy of Industrial Animal Factories*, which in 450 photographs and thirty essays provides an unprecedented view of concentrated animal feeding operations (CAFO), where increasing amounts of the world's meat, dairy, and seafood are produced.

Don't think that this level of animal abuse occurs just in third-world countries. Plenty of these torture-and-death houses exist in North America and Europe, producing most of the animal products that everyone—from the poor to the wealthy—consume each day. If you avail yourself of the informative resources that these compassionate and courageous folks have created, you will be shocked at the human indifference to farm animals' wills to live and the institutionalized cruelty perpetrated against these defenseless creatures whom we put on our dinner plates. As Kris Dannon, reviewing the aforementioned book, noted, *"What we once called a farm is now more a concentration camp than a farm."*

The scenes that confront one on such factory farms are torturous. Pigs are confined to gestation crates so small they can't even turn around. Ducks are force-fed with tubes jammed down their throats 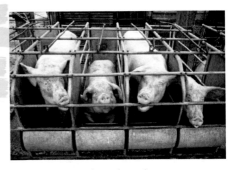 to fatten their livers to such grotesque sizes that their livers press on their lungs, making breathing so difficult that many die. Cows are painfully burned with searing-hot irons. Chickens' beaks are chopped off without anesthesia. Pigs have their genitals twisted from their bodies while they squeal in unimaginable agony. Dairy cows are artificially stimulated so they continue producing unnatural amounts of milk until they collapse in exhaustion. Cattle fear their death while lined up watching the animal in front of them be killed. Some reports indicate that up to one out of five cows are not stunned completely unconscious before being hoisted upside down into the air where their throats are slit and they die a slow, agonizing death.

Few know the interior lives of animals as well as Jane Goodall, the British primatologist, ethologist, anthropologist, and United Nations Messenger of Peace most famous for her forty-five-year study of the 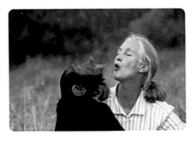 social and family interactions of wild chimpanzees. In The Inner World of Farm Animals, Goodall writes:

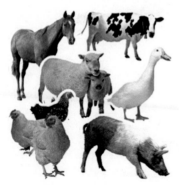

"Farm animals feel pleasure and sadness, excitement and resentment, depression, fear and pain. They are far more aware and intelligent than we ever imagined and, despite having been bred as domestic slaves, they are individual beings in their own right. As such they deserve our respect. And our help. Who will plead for them if we are silent?"

She challenges us: *"Thousands of people who say they 'love' animals sit down once or twice a day to enjoy the flesh of creatures who have been utterly deprived of everything that could make their lives worth living and who endured the awful suffering and the terror of the abattoirs [slaughter houses]—and the journey to get there—before finally leaving their miserable world, only too often after a painful death."*

Since animals are unable to communicate with us in a language that we understand, scientists have traditionally relied upon their behavioral observations to infer what animals may be thinking or feeling. Recent neurological studies conducted on alert dogs trained to lie still inside magnetic resonance imaging (MRI) machines have revealed startling results. Gregory Berns, a professor of neuroeconomics at Emory University and author of the 2013 book, *How Dogs Love Us: A Neuroscientist and His Adopted Dog Decode the Canine Brain*, has produced the first maps of dogs' brain activity. He writes:

We cannot ignore the striking similarity between dogs and humans in both the structure and function of a key brain region: the caudate nucleus. Rich in dopamine receptors, the caudate sits between the brainstem and the cortex. In humans, the caudate plays a key role in the anticipation of things we enjoy, like food, love and money. Caudate activation is so consistent that under the right circumstances, it can predict our preferences for food, music and even beauty. Many of the same things that activate the human caudate, which are associated with positive emotions, also activate the dog caudate.

Professor Berns explains that dogs' ability to experience love, attachment, and other positive emotions implies a level of sentience equivalent to a human child, which suggests that we need to rethink how we treat dogs. He writes, *"But now, using the MRI to push away the limits of behaviorism, we can no longer hide the evidence.* 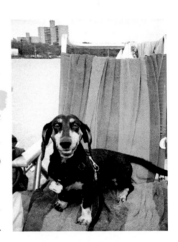 *Dogs, and probably many other animals (especially our closest primate relatives), seem to have emotions just like us. And this means we must reconsider their treatment as property."*

As more evidence begins trickling in about dogs and other animals' brain capacities being not dissimilar to those of humans, it is going to raise a host of uncomfortable questions about humans' treatment of animals, the worst being arguably the brutal conditions where they are forced to live and the horrific deaths they endure on the factory farms that disassemble their bodies for us to eat. Thankfully, there are a growing number of thoughtful consumers who are unwilling to continue turning a blind eye to this needless suffering of innocent animals. Among them is Danielle Licata, who poignantly describes in an essay in the Examiner.com what the farm animals we eat endure before their body parts are put on our plates.

Put Yourself in Their Hooves

A Second in the Life of a Factory Farm Animal

Imagine being taken from your mother at a very young age, never getting to feel her warm body or play with her in the sunshine. You are left to grieve and weep over the loss of a mother whom you will never know. Imagine being forced to live in a dark, cramped, feces infested room never knowing what fate awaits you. The smell is deadly, the diseases are prevalent, and the stress is high. Not having space to move your limbs causes high anxiety, so you chew on your skin to keep yourself sane. Imagine having hooks stuck in your weak body pulling you quickly along a conveyor belt. The pain is unbearable and your cries go unheard. You feel your own blood running down your body and the fear is so intense you urinate on yourself. Imagine having your life end with a cold knife to your throat or a skin boiling bath. Your last few images are your friends and kin suffering. Your last few breaths are cold and painful. Your last few thoughts are lonely and confusing.

© Danielle Licata

Any adult unfamiliar with these barbaric systemic practices of the factory farm animal industry is encouraged to go online and look at some of the undercover videos. Just search for 'factory farming videos' and you'll get results from a variety of organizations that have filmed what really goes on inside factory farms. The cruelty and suffering is enough to turn one's stomach. But we should not turn our eyes. We need to get the facts, and the animals deserve for us to see the truth. We must be their voices.

Is it any wonder why we renamed these poor animals' body parts and attractively packaged them so that at the grocery store all we see is steak ready to throw on the barbecue, with never a thought or image coming to mind of what that animal suffered? Who wants to acknowledge that the ground meat in our hands that we are forming into meatballs was an animal's muscle that animated his or her body, not unlike the muscles that animate our bodies?

Absent the risk of our own starvation, how can we justify taking animals' flesh, indeed their lives, from them? A psychologically healthy person cannot watch such documentary film footage of what really goes on inside industrial slaughter houses and not ask, is all of this pain, suffering, and death really necessary?

3

HOW WE CHOOSE WHAT TO EAT

Archeology tells us that our hunter-gatherer ancestors were omnivores and that once we domesticated our food sources, our diet included both plants and animals. Omnivores, with neither carnivore nor herbivore specializations for acquiring and processing food, are generalized opportunistic feeders who consume whatever is available to survive.

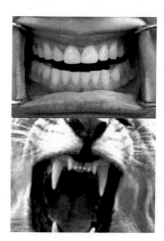

Scientists who have examined dental records have concluded that humans are more suited for a plant-based diet with little meat. Humans have only four meat-tearing canine teeth, as compared to carnivores such as lions, wolves, alligators, and sharks that have more. Humans' eight frontal incisor teeth are used to bite fruits and vegetables. The majority of our teeth are molars, which are ideal for grinding and crushing plants and seeds. Moreover, human saliva is alkaline and full of enzymes such as amylase that are highly effective in processing plants and carbohydrates. Carnivores, on the other hand, have mostly acidic saliva without amylase. In addition, human intestines are four times longer than we are tall, as compared to carnivores whose intestines average only two times their height. Our longer tract allows for more time to process the complex carbohydrates within plants, whereas carnivores' shorter tracts allow meat to pass quickly with less rot and putrefaction.

In short, humans are not preadapted to be either meat eaters or vegetarians, but are capable of being both. But although we can digest it if needed to avoid starving, animal flesh is not ideally suited for human consumption and is not needed in an omnivore's diet.

No doubt, cooked animal flesh tastes good. Over the course of civilization the perception developed that it was a more desirous food, though often limited to the wealthy who could afford it. Modern generations were raised on the idea that eating meat was necessary for optimal health. For example, people with iron-poor blood were often encouraged to eat red meat. Research has subsequently revealed that some of those assumptions were false. In fact, on a per calorie basis, dried beans and dark green leafy vegetables are better sources of iron.

For Americans, perhaps no single party is as responsible for our belief in the necessity of animal products in our diet as the US Department of Agriculture (USDA). For decades, the USDA published its Nutrition Guidelines to advise Americans about the foods that make up a healthy diet including, of course, the meat, poultry, eggs, and dairy products sold by the agricultural companies whose commercial interests it is the USDA's primary mission to advance. Prominent among its recommendations are some of the very foods that we now know can cause chronic inflammation and illness such as arteriosclerosis, diabetes, and cancer.

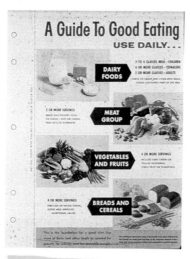

Not surprisingly, the cattle industry, pork producers, chicken factory farms, pâté purveyors, and others have a financial interest in keeping meat on our breakfast tables, lunch menus, and dinner plates. Because of this they spend millions of dollars each year to advertise their products and maintain the illusion that we need to eat what are, in fact, dead animal body parts and decaying flesh.

The truth is, we don't need to eat these products. Science tells us that it is not required for our nourishment and well-being. We can choose to not eat the animals and actually enhance our own health.

Many object that meat consumption has historically been an accepted part of the human diet, that killing animals is so widely viewed as normal, and that it is such an important and entrenched business practice that to expect people to change is unrealistic.

One can imagine similar arguments being made in the past against other social changes, such as slavery, upon which entire economies were built and livelihoods depended. Child labor was once considered necessary to support poor families until we agreed as compassionate people to develop charitable organizations and provide government assistance. Accepting dangerous working conditions was considered just part of the job until people rightly demanded passage of occupational safety regulations. The arc of human history bends toward raising our consciousness and changing practices that are harmful, unjust, or undignified.

Such changes, however disruptive to entrenched social practices, don't go unrewarded. Just ask American women who got the right to vote in 1920, less than one hundred years ago. It is hard to imagine today that what was once considered "normal" subservience of women to men went unchallenged for centuries. Generation after generation grudgingly accepted restrictions on women that we now find cringeworthy, not unlike how we've grown accustomed to eating meat, never giving a thought to the animal who suffered for our self-indulgence. Sometimes obvious injustice exists right under our noses, yet we smell nothing foul.

Today, as close as our local market, we see costumed evidence of the needless suffering of animals. In North America, it's mostly cows, pigs, chickens, turkeys, and ducks. In other countries, cows and ducks are sacred, but dogs and cats are eaten. Many of us love our dogs and cats, but think for a moment of our history with them. Who could have imagined their movement from outside our tribal campfires and into our yards, our homes, and more recently our hearts? These two species of animals, once considered merely of utilitarian value, now play enriching relational roles in our human lives. Who doesn't smile tenderly when seeing a veteran reunited with his beloved best friend after a long absence, when glimpsing a child hugging her fluffy kitty, or when encountering a blind man able to navigate a busy sidewalk thanks to the help of his trained seeing-eye dog? But consider: Pigs are known to have as much or more intelligence than some dogs. Cows mourn the absence of their calves. Chickens engage in self-validating behaviors. Elephants recognize the bones of their fallen comrades. Horses develop trusting relationships with humans. The more animal behaviorists spend time with animals, the more we learn about how much more complex are their interior lives than we ever imagined.

This all begs the question posed by, among others, Mercy For Animals, that we would be wise and compassionate to ask ourselves: "Why love one but eat the other?"

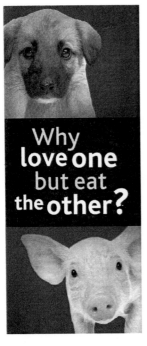

To mistake animals' limited communication ability as a lack of intelligence, emotions, or will to live because they don't have the physical apparatus humans have to form complex sounds into meaningful language that we understand: (1) does an injustice to the animals as our fellow sentient beings; (2) blinds us to the opportunity to develop dignified, respectful, even affectionate human–animal relationships; and (3) creates the disturbed illusion that animals are "things" of no concern to us, rather than "beings" whose care is entrusted to us.

We live in a relationship of stewardship that has been perverted by callousness and indifference. If we were more attentive, we would begin to appreciate the interior lives of our fellow creatures.

A posting on the website pinkjooz.com anecdotally describes the giving and receiving of affection among different species of animals to which any warm hearted human can relate.

We Hug and Kiss, What Do Animals Do?

When we see our loved ones and feel affectionate, we hug and kiss them. Or sometimes just a warm touch is enough. And sometimes you ruffle their hair to show you care. It is the same with animals. They too have feelings and are quite generous in showing it. But how do they do it? How do the animals show their love? What is their version of "hug n kiss"? Actually, each animal has their own way of expressing their love. Here are some of the extremely cute gestures animals use to show love:

1. Squirrels: To show love they sniff their partner's neck and entangle their tails.

2. Dogs: Dog's equivalent to kiss is touching nose. They also embrace each other by standing up on hind legs.

3. Bears: They roll on the ground while embracing each other.

4. Parrots: They rub their beaks together.

5. Chimpanzees: They do tongue kissing or what we humans called smooching!

6. Snails: It caresses its partner's antennae.

7. Cows: Cows kiss with lips and they are known to kiss for hours.

8. Rabbits: They scratch and do fisticuffs to show love.

9. Giraffes: They entwine their necks together.

10. Horses: They rub nose.

11. Swans: They entwine their necks and then rub their beaks.

12. Cats: Lick each other and sleep using each other's body as pillows.

13. Sea Lions: Suck on each other's ear flaps.

14. Lions: They head rub each other.

15. Deer: They kiss with lips and touch nose to show affection.

16. Owls: Kiss by tapping their beaks and cuddle by pressing up against each other

17. Snakes: They show love by touching its partner's tongue.

18. Penguins: Even humans "Penguin kiss" each other. They kiss by touching their beaks briefly to their partners.

© pinkjooz.com

Consider how animals can overcome their fear and develop relationships of trust with humans. Any equestrian will tell you that central to the human–horse relationship is the trust that the human tries to earn from the horse. Speaking in quiet tones, reinforcing with treats, and gradually moving from touching the horse's head to running one's hands all over the horse's body slowly earns the horse's trust that the rider is a friend and need not be feared. Many of us have experienced similar relationship-building after adopting a dog. Perhaps timid and fearful at first, especially if abused, a dog is smart enough to learn from our behavior whether we can be trusted. Indeed, one of the most gratifying human experiences is earning a once-fearful animal's trust.

Some of you may be familiar with Christian the lion who had been purchased in 1969 from Harrod's department store in London by two Australian men, Anthony Bourke and John Rendall, who created a den for him in the basement of their furniture store, played with him in the local churchyard and, as he grew larger, reintroduced him to the wild with the help of conservationist George Adamson at Kenya's Kora Natural Reserve.

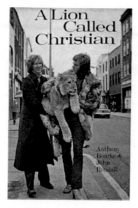 Most remarkable about this relationship is that a year later when the two men traveled back to Kenya to check on Christian's adjustment to life in the wild, Christian not only recognized them but leapt playfully into their arms, wrapped his front legs around their shoulders, and nuzzled their faces in a display of affection that shattered our understanding of the limits of human–lion interaction. The relationship was documented in the book *A Lion Called Christian* and in the film *Christian, The Lion at World's End*.

More recently, a South African game warden and his wife, Tonie and Shirley Joubert, rescued an orphaned one-day-old hippopotamus, Jessica, who has since become a family member with free reign of their property and home. Although Jessica spends time with other hippos, she considers the humans' home her home. She is able to open the front door and let herself into the kitchen where she sidles up to the counter to be fed, and at night she sleeps on a mattress on the floor, cuddled up with the family dog.

Closer to home in British Columbia, Canada, Mark Dumas adopted a six-week-old polar bear, the world's largest land predator.

Amazingly, Mr. Dumas and the polar bear became friends who now swim, frolic, and hug each other to show their mutual affection.

Slowly but surely some of our faulty assumptions about animals are giving way to greater understanding about their capacity to develop bonds not just within their own species, but across species, including with humans. Their relationships are based upon learning more about each other and gradually building mutual trust.

Just like people, animals are best known not in groups but as individuals. Each person and each animal has his or her unique personality, preferences, and pathos.

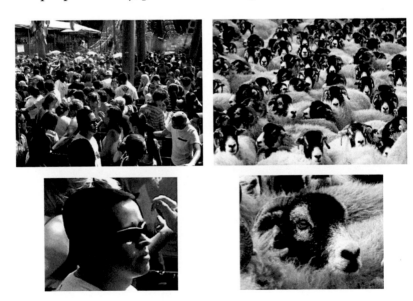

It's hard for us to relate personally to a crowd of people or animals, but spend time with just one person or just one animal and from that experience will emerge a relationship of budding familiarity. Sentient beings relate to one another, irrespective of species.

Each animal, whether on the farm or in the wild, seeks to preserve his or her own life, to frolic with kin and to care for offspring. All animals know how to enjoy their life—if we let them.

But should we? Should we leave animals to live their natural lives and stop confining, cutting, and cooking them?

This is where the decision of whether to eat the animals moves beyond the convenient illusion of simply being a dietary choice and into its authentic dimension of being a moral issue with existential consequences.

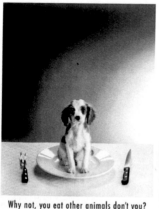

Why not, you eat other animals don't you?

THE VEGETARIAN SOCIETY **Y**

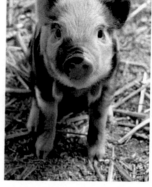

As uncomfortable as it may be for us to acknowledge to ourselves, there is no denying the harsh reality of the fates that await different animals simply because our human cultures have grown accustomed to eating some animals while loving others, in spite of the fact that there is no metaphysical or moral difference among them as sentient beings.

Whether an animal lives in a jungle, on a farm, or in a family home does not change the nature of the animal's sentience—its ability to feel, perceive, and experience its own subjectivity. As Mark Bekoff, Ph.D., wrote in June 2013 in *Psychology Today*, "We know that individuals of a wide variety of species experience emotions ranging from joy and happiness to deep sadness, grief, and PTSD, along with empathy, jealousy and resentment."

On July 7, 2012, a group of scientists at Cambridge University publicly proclaimed The Cambridge Declaration of Consciousness, writing:

> Convergent evidence indicates that nonhuman animals have the neuroanatomical, neurochemical, and neurophysiological substrates of conscious states along with the capacity to exhibit intentional behaviors. Consequently, the weight of evidence indicates that humans are not unique in possessing the neurological substrates that generate consciousness. Nonhuman animals, including all mammals and birds, and many other creatures, including octopuses, also possess these neurological substrates.

In other words, animals' subjective experience of their lives is not all that different than certain dimensions of our own. They fear the knife at their throat not unlike we do.

Factory farmed animals needlessly suffer and prematurely die because of our human denial—the psychological defense mechanism we use to reject what is real or true, despite overwhelming evidence to the contrary. For some of us it may be simple denial of unpleasant facts. The sterility of supermarket packaging certainly helps in this regard. Others may accept the reality of animal suffering but deny its seriousness. This is a convenient, self-serving rationalization. Still others may admit the horrors on factory farms, and appreciate the seriousness of animal suffering, but deny responsibility by blaming others who do the actual killing. The truth is, the direct connection from slaughterhouse to supermarket to supper table eliminates the possibility of absolving any of us of at least some responsibility.

> *"Anyone who says that life matters less to animals than it does to us has not held in his hands an animal fighting for its life. The whole being of the animal is thrown into that fight, without reserve."*
>
> Elisabeth Costello, in J.M. Coetzee's The Lives of Animals

4
THE MORAL DIMENSION OF EATING THE ANIMALS

Each year in the United States, we send to their death 150 million cattle, bison, sheep, hogs, and goats and nine billion chickens, turkeys, and ducks. In Canada, 650 million farm animals are killed annually. In the European Union, 300 million cattle, sheep, and pigs and an estimated four billion chickens have their lives prematurely ended. Raising those billions of animals to profit from their killings produces methane, a potent greenhouse gas that traps more heat than carbon dioxide. According to the United Nations, this industrial-scale animal production accounts for almost 18 percent of the world's climate change.

But even worse than the bloodletting of all of these animals and the pollution of our environment is that all of this livestock production and slaughter uses about 30 percent of the earth's land surface, land that could be used to grow more plants and grains for human consumption and help prevent the premature deaths of twenty million humans each year due to starvation and diseases related to malnutrition.

According to Dr. Richard Oppenlander, author of the 2011 book, *Comfortably Unaware*, 82 percent of the world's starving children live in countries where food is fed to animals that are killed and eaten by wealthier people in developed countries. One-fourth of all grain produced by developing countries is given to livestock in their own countries and elsewhere. While it would be simplistic to suggest that the complex problem of eradicating hunger could be solved by just giving poor people the grain otherwise fed to livestock, we do know that what wealthy countries choose to eat influences global resource use, food policies, foreign aid, and development projects.

Livestock production is a very inefficient and resource-depleting form of agriculture. Converting grains to animal flesh wastes most of the grain's protein and energy. Growing crops to feed livestock requires tremendous amounts of water and often leads to soil erosion.

Dr. Oppenlander notes that in certain resource-depleted areas of the Horn of Africa, where cattle occupy 44 percent of the land, farmers are able to produce two thousand to three thousand pounds of grain, vegetables, and fruit per acre for human consumption, but less than one hundred pounds of meat when that land is used for livestock. Here is a brief excerpt of his insightful analysis.

Animal Agriculture, Hunger and How to Feed a Growing Global Population

In a number of African countries, for instance, hunger and poverty form a complex cycle, each affecting the other and involving education, human health and social inequities, political instability, and depletion of natural resources. Food choices in the affected country as well as in other, more developed countries, significantly influence this cycle, touching each of the components. Of primary importance is the decision whether to eat animal- or plant-based foods.

We are producing enough grain globally to feed two times as many people as there are on earth. In 2011, there was a record harvest of grain in the world, with over 2.5 billion tons, but half of that was fed to animals in the meat and dairy industries. Seventy-seven percent of all coarse grains (corn, oats, sorghum, barley) and over 90 percent of all soy grown in the world was fed to livestock. Add to that the 30 percent food wasted from farm to table, and we see clearly that the difficulty is not *how* to produce enough food to feed the hungry but rather *where* all the food we produce is going.

Purely plant-based organic agricultural systems have been shown to be the most effective at long-term soil rebuilding, increasing yields in some districts by as much as 400 percent. Quite simply, many countries in Africa and in the Amazonian region that suffer from hunger raise cattle at the expense of their soil and other resources, while producing a fraction of the food they could if they converted to plant-based foods.

© Dr. Richard Oppenlander

Echoing the breadth of benefits of a plant-based diet as described by Dr. Oppenlander in his book, Dr. Neal Barnard, president of the Physicians Committee for Responsible Medicine, notes, "As vegan diets gain popularity across the country for a way to improve health and the welfare of animals, it's no secret that the environmental effects of this diet can have a positive effect on our planet."

And let's not forget about the amount of food we waste. According to the United Nations' food agency, one-third of the food produced for human consumption—1.43 billion tons—gets lost or wasted each year. In the United States, consumers waste 9 percent of what they order in restaurants, partly due to the trend of large portion sizes. The U.N. reports that simple measures such as better storage and reducing oversized portions would sharply reduce the amount of food wasted.

If we connect the dots, a pattern of consumption and waste begins to emerge. We in the developed world are becoming increasingly obese while those in the developing world go to bed hungry.

Pope Francis has weighed in on this from the high-level view of the developed world's focus on money and materialism. We devote great attention to, and personally anguish over, dips in the financial markets while we blithely accept human hunger as normal and largely ignore it. It isn't normal, and since taking office in March 2013, Pope Francis has conveyed his desire to see the world's 1.2 billion Roman Catholics defend the poor and practice more austerity.

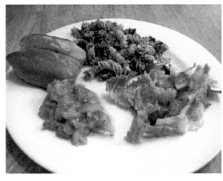

Since the nutritional adequacy of plant-based diets for all life stages has been scientifically established, there is no nutritional reason why we cannot forego eating the animals and, indeed, live even healthier, more energetic lives by eating vegetables, legumes, fruits, grains, seeds, and nuts grown from the earth with greater efficiency and yields, and less waste and resource depletion. It's good for us, good for our fellow human beings, good for the animals, and good for our environment.

After taking all of these benefits into account, it is admittedly conceivable that a person, irrespective of his or her faith, or lack thereof, could nonetheless remain:

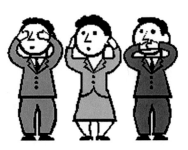

- Unconcerned about the cumulative negative impact of eating meat and animal-based food products upon his or her own and family's health;

- Uninterested in opportunities to produce more food to feed the world's poor;

- Indifferent to the needless pain, suffering, and premature deaths of innocent animals at human hands; and

- Apathetic about climate change's predicted damaging impact upon future generations.

In that case, upon what basis should that person still ask him- or herself, "Should I continue to eat meat?"

I believe that the question boils down to a simple moral decision: "If I can satisfy all of my nutritional requirements by eating a variety of vegetables, fruits, legumes, grains, nuts, and seeds, is it moral for me to continue eating meat, which I know promotes all of the aforementioned deleterious effects on people, animals, and our planet?"

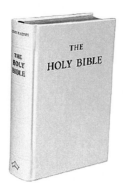

It's customary in grappling with moral challenges to examine one's spiritual beliefs. In the West, reference is often made to the Bible, where we find plenty of passages where God talks about His, and our, relationship with animals.

The Old Testament tells us that man was given dominion over the animals in Genesis 1:27-30:

> So God created man in his own image, in the image of God he created him; male and female he created them. And God blessed them. And God said to them, "Be fruitful and multiply and fill the earth and subdue it, and have dominion over the fish of the sea and over the birds of the heavens and over every living thing that moves on the earth." And God said, "Behold, I have given you every plant yielding seed that is on the face of all the earth, and every tree with seed in its fruit. You shall have them for food. And to every beast of the earth and to every bird of the heavens and to everything that creeps on the earth, everything that has the breath of life, I have given every green plant for food." And it was so.

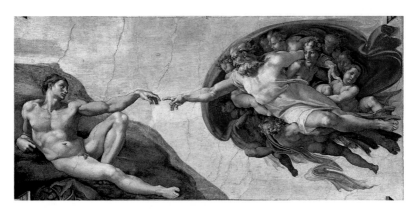

In the creation story we learn of man's divine source and image and his mandated stewardship over the animals, as well as the intention that man and animal alike were to eat plants and grains, not each other. For those who put little stock in the creation story's dietary directive, consider what science tell us.

Recall the American Dietetic Association's statement quoted in Chapter 1: "It is the position of the American Dietetic Association that appropriately planned vegetarian diets, including total vegetarian or vegan diets, are healthful, nutritionally adequate, and may provide health benefits in the prevention and treatment of certain diseases. Well-planned vegetarian diets are appropriate for individuals during all stages of the life cycle." Scientific research has validated the Bible's dietary prescriptive to eat plants and grains exclusively.

Later in the Scriptures we learn that the original sin of man's rebellion against God tainted the created order, which not only changed the once peaceful relationship among animals to that of hunter and prey, but also altered humans' relationship with animals, instilling fear of humans in the animals and granting humans limited permission to hunt and consume—if we can catch them. Animals remain important creations of God for whom he has care. After the flood, God mentions five times, "I will make a covenant with you and with all living creatures."

We read in Genesis 9:1-4:

> And God blessed Noah and his sons and said to them, "Be fruitful and multiply and fill the earth. The fear of

you and the dread of you shall be upon every beast of the earth and upon every bird of the heavens, upon everything that creeps on the ground and all the fish of the sea. Into your hand they are delivered. Every moving thing that lives shall be food for you. And as I gave you the green plants, I give you everything. But you shall not eat flesh with its life, that is, its blood."

Whereas humans and animals once lived together in peace, with neither human lust for animal flesh nor animal fear of humans, the relationship was irreparably damaged and corrupted with violence—animals attacking humans and humans hunting animals.

The limited permission to eat animal flesh granted after the flood is spelled out in the books of Leviticus and Deuteronomy that, among other things, describe how the Law of Moses makes dietary distinctions between animals that the Jewish people were and were not allowed to eat.

In the New Testament we know that Jesus ate broiled fish and served bread and fish to the hungry. Although there is no mention of Jesus eating meat, the Gospels do mention Jesus keeping three Passover feasts, meals where roast lamb, bitter herbs, and unleavened bread would have been served. Whether Jesus ate the lamb that was presumably served is unknown because the Scriptures are silent on this point.

It is worth noting that in the Nazareth of Jesus's time, meals were very simple and eaten only twice a day. They were primarily comprised of bread, legumes, oil, and fruit. Some of the Apostles made their living as fishermen, so we know that fish was prized as a food. According to Eric Eve, a New Testament scholar at Oxford University quoted in a May 23, 2005 BBC News story, "The staple diet of a Mediterranean peasant in Jesus' day would have been bread. Around Lake Tiberias, the Sea of Galilee, fish would also have been significant, though for peasants perhaps only in small quantities to provide a relish for the bread."

Occasionally, usually for feasts such as Passover, the flesh of land animals was consumed. Meat was a special food, and slaughtering an animal was a significant event. We're familiar with the parable of the prodigal son whose father was so overjoyed at his son's return home after a disappointing and lengthy absence that they feasted on a fatted calf.

According to God's law and Jesus's example, the eating of certain animal flesh was not forbidden, but was reserved for occasional consumption—in thanksgiving—during meals of special importance.

In the Bible God reminds us that the animals belong to him and in granting us dominion over them, he also gives us certain responsibilities to look after the animals with care and respect. Take, for example, Psalm 50:10: "For every beast of the forest is mine, the cattle on a thousand hills. I know all the birds of the hills, and all that moves in the field is mine." Another example is Proverbs 12:10: "Whoever is righteous has regard for the life of his beast, but the mercy of the wicked is cruel."

In Exodus 23:5 we learn that God expects us to care for people and animals: "If you see the donkey of one who hates you lying down under its burden, you shall refrain from leaving him with it; you shall rescue it with him."

In Exodus 23:12 God tells us to respect animals' needs as our own: "Six days you shall do your work, but on the seventh day you shall rest; that your ox and your donkey may have rest, and the son of your servant woman, and the alien, may be refreshed. In Exodus 23:3 and Deuteronomy 22:4 we read, "If you see an animal that is overburdened, you should lighten its load to help it."

The Scriptures even humble humans relative to the animals, as in Ecclesiastes 3:18-20:

> I said in my heart with regard to the children of man that God is testing them that they may see that they themselves are but beasts. For what happens to the children of man and what happens to the beasts is the same; as one dies, so dies the other. They all have the same breath, and man has no advantage over the beasts, for

all is vanity. All go to one place. All are from the dust, and to dust all return.

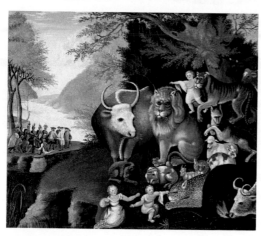

These are sober words that should inculcate within each of us a respect for life wherever we may find it. Presumably with such respect would come understanding that dominion over the animals does not mean the tyranny of treating innocent animals like condemned prisoners, abusing them, mutilating them, causing them needless suffering, preventing them from engaging in the behaviors natural to their species, and mindlessly slaughtering, skinning, and slicing them up in industrial-scale meat factories.

Although the Bible allows for sacrificing and eating animals, it's important to note that such permission was given *after* creation was marred by sin. God's original intention was that neither humans nor animals would eat flesh. In the Garden of Eden, before Adam and Eve disobeyed God, humans had dominion over the animals but didn't eat them. God instructed them to eat heartily of just the vegetation. Genesis 1:29: "And God said, 'See, I have given you every herb that yields seeds which is on the face of all the earth, and every tree whose fruit yields seed; to you it shall be food.'"

Isaiah, in prophesying about the future Messianic kingdom, gave a clear and inspiring description of the harmony of paradise shared even among the carnivorous animals and their natural prey. Isaiah 11:6–9:

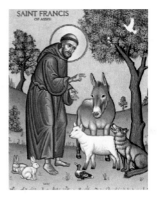

The wolf shall dwell with the lamb, and the leopard shall lie down with the young goat, and the calf and the lion and the fattened calf together; and a little child shall lead them. The cow and the bear shall graze; their young shall lie down together; and the lion shall eat straw like the ox. The nursing child shall play over the hole of the cobra, and the weaned child shall put his hand on the adder's den. They shall not hurt or destroy in all my holy mountain; for the earth shall be full of the knowledge of the Lord as the waters cover the sea.

This is a compelling picture of our eternal destiny that we are graced with glimpses of during our temporal lives. Consider how good we feel when we're able to overcome animals' apprehensions and they succumb to our entreaties and treats and finally trust us. Dean Ohlman, resident ethicist of Restoring Eden, Christians for Environmental Stewardship, writes about the peaceable kingdom, saying "It may be an indication that in the heart of every person is a longing for the harmony that once reigned in the Garden of Eden."

Many across time and cultures champion the cause of animals. Buddha, the fourth century BC sage, said: "All beings tremble before violence. All fear death. All love life. See yourself in others. Then whom can you hurt? What harm can you do?"

In the Laws of Manu, a Hindu religious text circa 1500 BC, we read,

> Meat cannot be obtained without injury to animals, and the slaughter of animals obstructs the way to Heaven; let him therefore shun the use of meat... He who does not eat meat becomes dear to men, and will not be tormented by diseases. He who permits the slaughter of an animal, who kills it, he who cuts it up, he who buys or sells meat, he who cooks it, he who serves it up, and he who eats it, are all slayers. There is no greater sinner than that man who seeks to increase the bulk of his own flesh by the flesh of other beings.

Consider what Pythagoras, the Greek mathematician and philosopher (c.570–495 BC), wrote:

> Alas, what wickedness to swallow flesh into our own flesh, to fatten our greedy bodies by cramming in other bodies, to have one living creature fed by the death of another! You cannot appease the hungry cravings of your wicked, gluttonous

stomachs except by destroying some other life. As long as man continues to be the ruthless destroyer of lower living beings he will never know health or peace. For as long as men massacre animals, they will kill each other. Indeed, he who sows the seed of murder and pain cannot reap joy and love.

Read Plutarch, the first century chronicler of Roman generals and emperors (c.46–120 AD). His words from centuries ago are just as relevant today in our age of unsurpassed animal carnage in industrial scale factory farms.

Can you really ask what reason Pythagoras had for abstaining from flesh? For my part I rather wonder both by what accident and in what state of soul or mind the first man did so, touched his mouth to gore and brought his lips to the flesh of a dead creature, he who set forth tables of dead, stale bodies and ventured to call food and nourishment the parts that had a little before bellowed and cried, moved and lived. How could his eyes endure the slaughter when throats were slit and hides flayed and limbs torn from limb? How could his nose endure the stench? How was it that the pollution did not turn away his taste, which made contact with the sores of others and sucked juices and serums from mortal wounds?

…The obligations of law and equity reach only to mankind, but kindness and benevolence should be extended to the creatures of every species, and these will flow from the breast of a true man, in streams that issue from the living fountain. Man makes use of flesh not out of want and necessity, see ing that he has the liberty to make his choice of herbs and fruits, the plenty of which is inexhaustible; but out of luxury, and being cloyed with necessaries, he seeks after impure and inconvenient diet, purchased by the slaughter of living beasts; by showing himself more cruel than the most savage of wild beasts...were it only to learn benevolence to human kind, we should be merciful to other creatures...

It is certainly not lions and wolves that we eat out of self-defense; on the contrary, we ignore these and slaughter harmless, tame creatures without stings or teeth to harm us, creatures that, I swear, Nature appears to have produced for the sake of their beauty and grace. But nothing abashed us, not the flower-like tinting of the flesh, not the persuasiveness of the harmonious voice, not the cleanliness of their habits or the unusual intelligence that may be found in the poor wretches. No, for the sake of a little flesh we deprive them of sun, of light, of the duration of life to which they are entitled by birth and being...Why do you belie the earth, as if it were unable to feed and nourish you? Does it not shame you to mingle murder and blood with her beneficent fruits? Other carnivores you call savage and ferocious—lions and tigers and serpents—while yourselves come behind them in no species of barbarity. And yet for them murder is the only means of sustenance! Whereas to you it is superfluous luxury and crime!

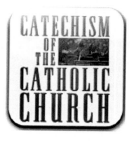

For Christians, the Catechism of the Catholic Church provides valuable insights that can inform our posture toward the animals whom God has placed to live among us during our temporal journey on Earth. From section 2415: "Use of the mineral, vegetable, and animal resources of the universe cannot be divorced from respect for moral imperatives. Man's dominion over inanimate and other living beings granted by the Creator is not absolute; it is limited by concern for the quality of life of his neighbor, including generations to come; it requires a religious respect for the integrity of creation." Section 2416: "Animals are God's creatures. He surrounds them with his providential care. By their mere existence they bless him and give him glory. Thus men owe them kindness."

Of particular note is that more is expected of us than just not causing animals needless suffering and premature death. What we fail to do that we should do (what Catholics call sins of *omission*) is as important as what we do that we shouldn't (sins of *commission*). Not causing animals harm is not enough. We must also be kind to them, not because it's good for us, but because they are creatures of God. Our relationship with God involves a duty of kindness toward animals.

It should not be lost on those familiar with the Scriptures that Jesus was born in a manger, a trough for animal feed, and 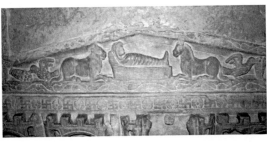 in an allusion to Isaiah we read that animals were chosen by God to also be witnesses to the Savior's birth—"the ox knoweth his owner, and the ass his master's crib"—a relationship depicted in this fourth-century sarcophagus showing an ox and a donkey surrounding the infant Jesus.

To develop a deeper appreciation of animals, it may be helpful to ask ourselves from where do we think the animals came? Isn't it obvious that they came from the same source as us? We didn't create ourselves anymore than we created the animals. For those who believe, the animals, like us, are the handiwork of God. He ideated them, just as he ideated us. He formed them, male and female, just as he formed us, male and female. He filled them with the breath of life—*nephesh* in Hebrew—just as he filled us. He imbued them with the power to procreate and to raise their offspring just like He did us. He put them on this earth to live out their natural lives just as he put us here.

Animals are placed in our custody, and we have a responsibility of stewardship to care for them. But the animals belong to God, no less than we belong to God. He gave us the animals as a gift, not to possess but to enrich our lives. If we make the effort, we will increasingly understand each other. The problem is that few try. In our modernity, we seem more intrigued with inanimate objects powered by electricity than by fellow creatures who breathe the same air, share the same origin, and face the same temporal destiny as us. All of our bodies age and die. Human sensitivities may be served by burying animal corpses in different locales than human corpses, but we are all buried in the same earth.

God loves the animals just as he loves us. Our promised eternal life, in which some have hope and many have faith, will be shared with animals, not just generally as we read before in Isaiah ("The wolf shall dwell with the lamb...") but with the same specificity as our human beloveds. The Bible is silent on whether animals have souls, but we know that God's mercy has no limit. If our happiness in heaven need include the animals for whom we developed affection, who can say they won't be there? With God all things are possible.

> ### Prayer of St. Basil the Great (329–359), Doctor of the Church
>
> The earth is the Lord's and the fullness thereof, Oh, God, enlarge within us the sense of fellowship with all living things, our brothers the animals to whom you gave the earth as their home in common with us. We remember with shame that in the past we have exercised the high dominion of man with ruthless cruelty so that the voice of the earth, which should have gone up to you in song, has been a groan of travail. May we realize that they live not for us alone but for themselves and for you and that they love the sweetness of life.

5

LEGAL BUT NEITHER LOVING NOR LOGICAL

Notwithstanding that God originally intended that we not eat the animals, and that His vision of our future paradise involves no consumption of animals, one consequence of the original sin that tore the fabric of creation is that, during our temporary sojourn here on this beautiful but now imperfect earth, killing and eating animals is legally permissible, however much it may not be preferred.

Christians, and those who admire Judeo-Christian values, understand that we are to be *in* the world but not *of* the world, meaning that we are to live robust lives not by the world's values but by God's values.

Jesus taught that love is a nobler motivator than the law in informing our decisions and guiding our actions. That being the case, we are called to live our lives believing in, working toward, and hoping for the Kingdom of God where our relationship with God finds its intended intimacy, our relationships with people are authentically harmonious, and our relationships with animals are transformed from fear and violence to peace and affection.

If you have any doubts about your soul's eternal calling to love, consider how the beauty of acting out of love outshines simply complying with the law. Think about how you feel when touching a goat at a petting zoo, feeding a carrot to a horse, throwing crumbs to swimming 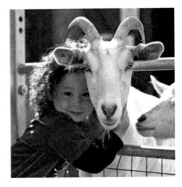 swans, or listening to a cow moo. Or think about when you're gazing at geese flying in formation, admiring the handsome face of a lion, laughing at the antics of chimps at play, or watching a paddling of ducks cross your path. You smile. You're amused. You feel good.

Now how would you feel if you were invited to engage in such activities as slitting a cow's throat, chopping off the head of a turkey, or skinning a lamb?

Most folks would cringe and smartly beg off the invitation. Why? Because we don't want to do harm. Rightly so and no one needs to teach us that. It is in the DNA of our humanity to care rather than to be cruel. Though we are capable of both, it is humans' natural default position, indeed our calling, to kindness, not killing. Kindness comes naturally and blossoms if we encourage it. Cruelty is a perversion of our natures, and all but the pathological would agree that it should be discouraged. Sadly, what goes on every day in the slaughterhouses that supply our supermarkets and butcher shops is nothing less than calculated cruelty and needless killing. It needs to stop.

If most of us are averse to directly engaging in such bloody, stomach-wrenching activities as slaughtering animals ourselves, why do we let others do it on our behalf? Don't we bear some culpability for the senseless suffering and premature deaths that butchers are going to visit upon those animals whom we'd prefer not to see with our eyes, yet are willing to eat with our mouths? If it is painful for us to even watch, imagine how painful it must be for each animal to endure.

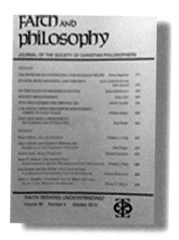

Faith and Philosophy Volume 15, Issue 2, April 1998 Reflections on the 20th Anniversary of the Society of Christian Philosophers Andrew Tardiff, Pages 210–22

With knowledge comes responsibility, and our highest responsibility is to act out of love. Confining, killing, and cooking animals when we have other foods to fully nourish our bodies may be legal, but it is not loving. What message do we send our children when we kill the animals for whom they develop affection?

Is it even logical for Christians to continue to kill God's animals? Can philosophical reasoning illuminate our thinking?

Over a decade ago Andrew Tardiff wrote a very compelling case that has not received the attention it deserves. In *Faith and Philosophy* he describes "A Catholic Case for Vegetarianism" that is not built upon Church teachings but upon logic, neither rejecting any Catholic teachings nor embracing anything the Church rejects. He starts by noting that in the Church's understanding of the development of doctrine, the Church recognizes that the truths of faith and morality deepen over time. Moral truths are unchanging, but our understanding of their implications is revealed over time as circumstances change. In other words, we are looking at new applications. Not just Catholics but all Christians and people of good will can find common ground here.

Tardiff appeals to the logic laid out by St. Thomas Aquinas: "An act may be rendered unlawful if it be out of proportion to the end." Out of proportion is understood to mean that if one good is brought about and another good is destroyed, the good destroyed must not have been greater than the good that was brought about. It is also understood to mean that, 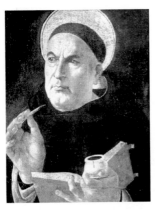 even if the good destroyed did not outweigh the good created, the act would still be unlawful if the good could have been created with less destruction. St. Thomas uses as an example being in a situation where we are about to be fatally attacked. If we need only injure, rather than kill, the offender to ward off the attack, we are morally justified in injuring but not in killing. The principle of proportionate good is one that we can apply in many areas of our lives.

St. Thomas held that all created things are ontically (existentially) good, including animals. He posits animals within a hierarchy of the created order.

> There exists...an operation of the soul which so far exceeds corporeal nature that it is not even performed by any corporeal organ; and such is the operation of the rational soul. *Below this*, there is another operation of the soul, which is indeed performed through a corporeal organ, but not through a corporeal quality; and this is the operation of the sensitive soul...*The lowest* of the operations of the soul is that which is performed by a corporeal organ, and by virtue of a corporeal quality...Such is the operation of the vegetative soul.

Humans are existentially higher than animals, and animals are higher than plants. The difference is not one of degree but one of kind. St. Thomas maintains that animals can do things that plants cannot do. Tardiff writes, "Leave aside their ability to move from place to place, and focus on the fact that animals can feel and perceive and remember. These abilities may be common, but that fact should not blind us to their high ontic status." He goes on to ask how an animal can possess another as an object of perception without itself being a subject: "Are not these inner life experiences of animals as private as they are for humans? And isn't what is true about perception also true about sensation and memory? How can there be a memory without someone remembering?" He goes on to state, "The step from the plant to the animal is at least the step from nonconscious to the conscious, from the amental to mind. Perhaps it is also the step from 'something' to 'someone.'"

When it comes to choosing whether to feed ourselves by either harvesting vegetables or slaughtering animals, the choice is not trivial. It is the difference between a conscious being with perception, sensation, relationships, and memory and a plant, which possesses none of those qualities. To eat protein-rich beans is to eat *something*. To eat protein-rich ground animal muscle requires killing

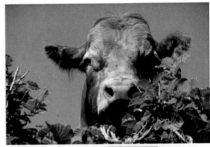
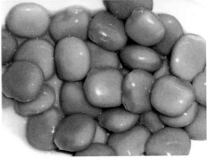

someone. Tardiff succinctly describes the consequence of St. Thomas's logic when he writes, "Simply stated, whenever a person can serve his ends by killing plants instead of animals, then he may not kill animals since, as ontically superior to plants, doing so in those circumstances would constitute more than necessary violence."

It's hard to argue with his logic. Of course, the argument depends upon two prior conditions, namely, the nutritional adequacy of diets not containing animal flesh, and the practical availability in adequate supply of vegetarian fare year-round. We already ascertained that from the contributions of science we now have the knowledge that a properly planned vegetarian diet not only is adequate for all life stages, but also results in better human health outcomes. The second condition depends upon particular circumstances that may vary for each individual. Those of us living in developed countries have convenient access to an abundance of the vegetables, fruits, legumes, grains, nuts, and seeds that comprise a nutritionally adequate diet. The same cannot be said for many people living in developing countries, or those without access to modern supermarkets, as is the case in many poor urban and rural neighborhoods.

For those of us fortunate enough to have nonanimal food sources readily available that can adequately nourish us, it's clear that killing an animal under these circumstances creates disproportionate destruction and is, therefore, not morally defensible. For those living in environments without ready access to adequately nutritious vegetarian sources, killing an animal to provide life-sustaining nourishment not otherwise available would do greater good than harm.

It is interesting to note, however, that it is precisely in the developed world with plenty of access to plant-based food sources that we see the greatest per capita consumption of meat—exactly opposite of what the principle of proportionate good would justify.

If you compare the meat consumption map on top with the GDP per capita map beneath it, the correlation is unmistakable.

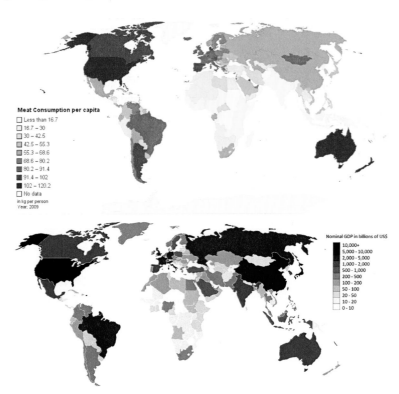

Asya Pereltsvaig makes this point in the article "Global Geography of Meat Consumption." The developed countries, whose populations have easy access to a whole cornucopia of food choices, are the biggest animal eaters, even though their meat consumption is not necessary since they are supplied year-round with plentiful, nutritious vegetarian fare.

Global Geography of Meat Consumption

By Asya Pereltsvaig

It is often suggested that the levels of meat consumption correlate with the overall economic development of a given country. A juxtaposition of the meat consumption map and the GDP per capita map confirms such a correlation: people in richer countries can afford to consume more meat than those in poorer countries. However, discrepancies here are instructive as well. For example, Brazilians and Venezuelans consume far more meat than would be expected on the basis of per capita GDP. Similarly, Gabon in central Africa consumes more meat than would be expected, as does Mongolia, where meat has always constituted a significant part of the diet. Turks, Romanians, and Belarusians too eat more meat than might be assumed on the basis of their GDP levels. Exceptions to the GDP/meat consumption correlation can be found in the opposite direction as well, with three clusters worldwide. First, relatively well-off South Africa and Botswana consume little meat. Second, Libya and Oman both rank high in terms of GDP, but have limited meat consumption; the wealth in those countries comes primarily from oil production and export and is therefore distributed quite unevenly, and the few extremely rich people can only eat so much meat. Finally, a significant number of countries with a high GDP but low levels of meat consumption can be found in East and Southeast Asia. In particular, Japan, South Korea, Malaysia, Singapore, and Taiwan consume less meat than would be expected based on their GDP.

© Asya Pereltsvaig, GeoCurrents

As noted earlier, it's not a coincidence that the populations in the animal-eating developed world are suffering from greater levels of obesity, diabetes, and other chronic illnesses.

We also now know that the destruction of that which is good is not limited to just the suffering and premature deaths of the animals. The quest for more and cheaper meat has intensified livestock production to an industrial scale that utilizes vast quantities of fertilizers and pesticides that cause dangerous levels of water and air pollution that damage human health. According to the UN Environmental Programme, the run-off from these chemicals is creating dead zones in the seas, causing toxic algal blooms, killing fish, and threatening amphibians and ecosystems.

What about bodily pleasure? Let's face it, cooked animal flesh tastes good. Bodily pleasure is, in and of itself, a good in life. But the pleasure of eating is not sacrificed in switching from an animal-based to a plant-based diet, since there are plenty of delicious vegetarian foods. All one is doing is merely sub-stituting some flavors in favor of other flavors, which is hard-ly a sacrifice. Tardiff uses a relevant example: "Consider the analogy of recreation. To ask a person to forego all recreation would be serious, almost inhuman. But to ask that he give up certain specific forms of recreation, like poker or basketball, would not. Such a person can easily lead a normal human life."

Those who are allergic to peanuts or strawberries, or who can't digest wheat gluten or dairy foods, or who prefer to avoid any variety of particular foods may not experience the flavors those specific foods can impart, but their palates are more than satis-fied with the bountiful alternatives that they can safely, comfort-ably, and enjoyably consume.

Tardiff deftly describes the Thomistic distinction between a hu-man act and the act of a human:

> Tasting the flavor of an animal is not a human pleasure, but merely the pleasure of a human. It does not require any specifically human faculties, but only animal ones. (The "rational" in "rational animal" does not figure in, only the "animal" does, since a dog, for example, certain-ly experiences the pleasure of meat in a comparable way.) The pleasure of eating meat is more accurately described as only an animal pleasure that a human has.

The implication is that, since an animal pleasure it not worth an animal's life, it is not proportionate to kill an animal for the pleasure of eating it. There are plenty of pleasurable-tasting plant-based foods to satisfy the human act of eating and nourishing ourselves.

But what about the special occasions, those feasts involving the consumption of particular animals—the succulent ham at Easter, the plump turkey at Thanksgiving, the juicy hamburger on the Fourth of July? Rather than making these wonderful social events dependent upon the killing of sentient creatures—which is not exactly conducive to conviviality—wouldn't we be encouraging more joy if we left the dead animal carcasses off the table and instead feasted on tasty vegetables, exotically spiced legumes, richly flavored grains, and sweet, delectable fruits?

Making such a change would enable us to enjoy different foods, taste new flavors, learn more about nutrition, promote our family's health, and rejoice with not a pang of guilt 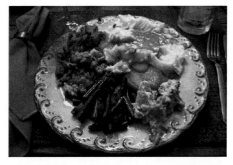 since neither turkey nor duck, chicken nor cow, pig nor lamb, had to be slaughtered in order for us to enjoy a feast with family and friends.

So let's see where we are. If (A) animals are of a wholly different order than plants, indeed *sentient someones*, not *nonconscious somethings*; and (B) under the circumstances of having adequately nutritious vegetarian fare readily available all year, it would do disproportionately more harm than good to kill the animals; and (C) the distinctly human acts that we are entitled to can be engaged in without causing the premature deaths of other creatures, what logical rationale are we left with to justify animal slaughter?

One could argue on a socio-economic level that factory farming is such a large industry upon which many businesses survive and employees depend for their livelihoods and is so integrated into our economy that it would be too disruptive for people en masse to stop buying animal flesh and to adopt a plant-based diet.

No doubt, the switch would have consequences, but those consequences needn't be feared because they would be good, indeed, disproportionately good.

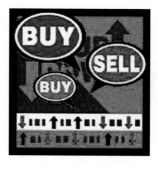

We are all not just free moral agents, but also consumers whose decisions about what we wish to purchase influence the enterprises that supply goods and services in the marketplace. Each of us needs to eat, so if we start buying more vegetables, legumes, grains, fruits, nuts, and seeds, and less ground chuck, chicken breasts, pork chops, venison, chateaubriand, and pâté, the agricultural industry will grow and harvest more plant foods and raise and slaughter fewer animals. Most elegantly within the capitalist economies, supply and demand will find the right balance so that our store shelves will continue to be stocked with the foods that our changing palates desire.

Agricultural resources that are inefficiently deployed for livestock production and slaughter would be more efficiently utilized for the growing and harvesting of food grown in and on the earth, making better use of limited farmland with less negative impact upon the environment. It would also provide less physically dangerous and psychically damaging jobs for farm workers who could return home after a hard day's work with just dirt, rather than blood, on their hands.

Transportation and distribution networks would still be required. Marketing and sales channels would be no less utilized. And shoppers would be able to feed their families healthier foods. Who knows, we might actually begin to see informative advertisements for real foods touting their nutritional advantages for our health as much as their taste, instead of the current commercials pitching food-like products whose pretty packaging masks a host of artificial ingredients.

As demand grows, competition could create opportunities for agricultural companies to better differentiate their products and generate brand loyalty, not unlike some fruit producers, such as Chiquita® with bananas and Dole® with pineapples, and some frozen vegetables producers, such as Green Giant® and Birds Eye®.

I believe that it is only a matter of time before the growing demand for organic foods, nutritional supplements, and healthier life-styles will usher in a growing distaste for slaughtered animal meat products. We already see the trend emerging in the grow-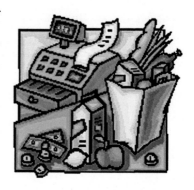ing popularity of vegetarian and vegan restaurants not just in major cities but in bedroom communities and sleepy suburbs, and the slow but steadily growing refrigerated shelf space in our supermarkets being allocated to vegan and vegetarian food products.

As more consumers are convinced of the advantages of eliminating animal flesh and eating a plant-based diet, there will still be plenty of money for agricultural companies to make, but without compromising human health, causing animal suffering, or generating needless environmental damage.

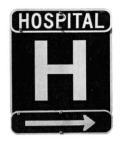 Even more, the strain on our healthcare system would be lessened as obesity, heart disease, diabetes, cancer, and other chronic illnesses would decline as diets get healthier. This would enable our medical practitioners to focus on less costly preventive medicine throughout the course of our longer lives, rather than diverting so many of our healthcare dollars to expensive clinical interventions for many conditions that erupt in middle and older age and that could have been reduced in intensity, or prevented altogether, by dietary changes.

It's surprising that our legislators in Washington, DC have not paid more attention in their sometimes-acrimonious debates about healthcare spending and health insurance coverage to the positive influence and impact that a meat-free foodstyle would have on the health of our bodies and budgets.

Agricultural businesses, by changing their product mix and means of production, would still be able to make handsome profits on us consumers.

 One exception, of course, might be the pharmaceutical companies, since there would be fewer animals to fill with anti-biotics and fewer humans needing choles-terol-lowering statins. But that would be a

small price to pay for a healthier population—a disproportionate good.

The logical outcomes of continuing to consume animal flesh are the slow but sure deterioration of our human health, the overuse of limited fertile land and water that could otherwise be used to raise vegetarian food for the malnourished, the further pollution of our environment, and the continued needless suffering and bloody deaths of millions of innocent, perceiving, sensing, remembering, and relational creatures, creatures who take the same breath of life as each of us.

The logical alternative is to stop eating the animals and expand our appreciation of them beyond their utilitarian value to us to their inherent existential value to themselves, to their familial value to their kin, to their relational value to us humans, and to their eternal value to God.

> "If everyone were to adopt a whole-food, plant-based diet, I really believe we could cut health care costs by 70 to 80 percent."
>
> —T. Colin Campbell, Ph.D., coauthor of *The China Study*, described by *The New York Times* as "the most comprehensive large study ever undertaken of the relationship between diet and the risk of developing disease."

6
A WEALTH OF WISDOM

The idea of not eating the animals is neither new nor culturally limited. Many intelligent people from different countries, time periods, and walks of life have tried to raise awareness of the plight of innocent animals needlessly suffering at human hands and of the associated human health consequences.

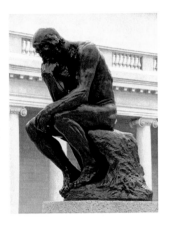

In this chapter, I invite you to read quotes from some of these astute individuals, courtesy of the thoughtful, humble soul behind the website all-creation.franciscan-anglican.com, which could very well contain the most extensive collection of quotes on this topic. One cannot read the words of these sensible and sensitive souls of great accomplishment and not hear the universality of their appeal, which crosses time, geography, and cultures. We would do well to embrace their wise counsel in order that our minds may be opened and our hearts moved.

Leonardo da Vinci (1452–1519), Renaissance painter, sculptor, architect, mathematician, engineer, inventor, and writer whom many consider the epitome of the humanist ideal

"I have since an early age adjured the use of meat, and the time will come when men such as I will look upon the murder of animals as they now look upon the murder of men. Truly man is the king of beasts, for his brutality exceeds them. We live by the death of others. We are burial places!"

Benjamin Franklin (1706–1790), one of the Founding Fathers of the United States, a scientist, statesman, and major figure in the American Enlightenment

"My refusing to eat flesh occasioned an inconveniency, and I was frequently chided for my singularity, but, with this lighter repast, I made the greater progress, for greater clearness of head and quicker comprehension. Flesh eating is unprovoked murder."

Dr. William Roberts, editor of *The American Journal of Cardiology*

"When we kill the animals to eat them, they end up killing us because their flesh, which contains cholesterol and saturated fat, was never intended for human beings."

John Jacques Rousseau (1712–1778), French philosopher, writer, and composer whose political philosophy influenced the French Revolution

"The animals you eat are not those who devour others; you do not eat the carnivorous beasts, you take them as your pattern. You only hunger after sweet and gentle creatures who harm no one, which follow you, serve you, and are devoured by you as the reward of their service."

Vaslav Nijinsky (1888–1950), famous Russian dancer and choreographer

"I do not like eating meat because I have seen lambs and pigs killed. I saw and felt their pain. They felt the approaching death. I could not bear it. I cried like a child. I ran up a hill and could not breathe. I felt that I was choking. I felt the death of the lamb."

Dr. Ashley Montagu (1905–1999), Chair of Anthropology, Rutgers University and author of *The Elephant Man*

"The indifference, callousness and contempt that so many people exhibit toward animals is evil first because it results in the great suffering of animals, and second because it results in an incalculably great impoverishment of the human spirit."

Matthew Scully, American author, journalist, and presidential speechwriter

"Factory farming isn't just killing: It is negation, a complete denial of the animal as a living being with his or her own needs and nature. It is not the worst evil we can do, but it is the worst evil we can do to them."

Isaac Singer (1904–1991), author of the first Yiddish book to win the Nobel Prize in literature

"When a human being kills an animal for food, he is neglecting his own hunger for justice. Man prays for mercy, but is unwilling to extend it to others. Why then should man expect mercy from God? It is unfair to expect something that you are not willing to give."

"As often as Herman had witnessed the slaughter of animals and fish, he always had the same thought: in their behaviour toward creatures, all men were Nazis. Human beings see oppression vividly when they're the victims. Otherwise they victimize blindly and without a thought."

"People often say that humans have always eaten animals, as if this is a justification for continuing the practice. According to this logic, we should not try to prevent people from murdering other people, since this has also been done since the earliest of times."

"There will be no justice as long as man will stand with a knife or with a gun and destroy those who are weaker than he is."

Tenzin Gyatso, Fourteenth Dalai Lama, leader of Tibetan Buddhism, and Nobel Peace Prize winner

"I do not see any reason why animals should be slaughtered to serve as human diet when there are so many substitutes. After all, man can live without meat. It is only some carnivorous animals that have to subsist on flesh. Killing animals for sport, for pleasure, for adventures, and for hides and furs is a phenomenon which is at once disgusting and distressing. There is no justification in indulging in such acts of brutality. In our approach to life, be it pragmatic or otherwise, the ultimate truth that confronts us squarely and unmistakably is the desire for peace, security and happiness. Different forms of life in different aspects of existence make up the teeming denizens of this earth of ours. And, no matter whether they belong to the higher group as human beings or to the lower group, the animals, all beings primarily seek peace, comfort and security. Life is as dear to a mute creature as it is to a man. Just as one wants happiness and fears pain, just as one wants to live and not to die, so do other creatures."

General Bramwell Booth (1829–1912), Founder of the Salvation Army

"The awful cruelty and terror to which tens of thousands of animals killed for human food are subjected in traveling long distances by ship and rail and road to the slaughterhouses of the world. God disapproves of all cruelty...whether to man or beast. The occupation of slaughtering animals is brutalizing to those who are required to do the work...I believe this matter is well worthy of the serious consideration of Christian leaders."

Count Leo Tolstoy (1828–1910), Russian author, philosopher, and theologian

"'Thou shalt not kill' does not apply to murder of one's own kind only, but to all living beings; and this Commandment was inscribed in the human breast long before it was proclaimed from Sinai."

"If he be really and seriously seeking to live a good life, the first thing from which he will abstain will always be the use of animal food, because...its use is simply immoral, as it involves the performance of an act which is contrary to the moral feeling—killing."

"As long as there are slaughterhouses, there will be battlefields."

"A man can live and be healthy without killing animals for food; therefore, if he eats meat, he participates in taking animal life merely for the sake of his appetite. And to act so is immoral. If a man aspires toward a righteous life, his first act of abstinence is from injury to animals."

Rt. Rev. Dr. John Baker (1928-2014), former Chaplain to the British House of Commons

"It is in the battery shed that we find the parallel with Auschwitz... To shut your mind, heart and imagination from the sufferings of others is to begin slowly, but inexorably, to die. Those Christians who close their minds and hearts to the cause of animal welfare, and the evils it seeks to combat, are ignoring the Fundamental spiritual teachings of Christ himself."

"Yet saddest of all fates, surely, is to have lost that sense of the holiness of life altogether; that we commit the blasphemy of bringing thousands of lives to a cruel and terrifying death or of making those lives a living death—and feel nothing."

Dr. Dean Ornish, Clinical Professor of Medicine, University of California San Francisco Medical School, and Physician to President Bill Clinton

"I don't understand why asking people to eat a well-balanced vegetarian diet is considered drastic, while it is medically conservative to cut people open and put them on cholesterol-lowering drugs for the rest of their lives."

Albert Einstein (1879–1955) German-born Nobel Prize-winning physicist

"Nothing will benefit human health and increase chances for survival of life on earth as much as the evolution to a vegetarian diet. It is my view that the vegetarian manner of living by its purely physical effect on the human temperament would most beneficially influence the lot of mankind."

"A human being is a part of the whole, called by us the 'Universe,' a part limited in time and space. He experiences himself, his thoughts and feelings, as something separate from the rest—a kind of optical delusion of his consciousness.

"This delusion is a kind of prison for us, restricting us to our personal desires and to affection for a few persons nearest to us. Our task must be to free ourselves from this prison by widening our circle of compassion to embrace all living creatures and the whole of nature in its beauty. Nobody is able to achieve this completely, but the striving for such achievement is in itself a part of the liberation and a foundation for inner security."

Fyodor Dostoyevsky (1821–1881), Russian novelist and philosopher

"Love animals: God has given them the rudiments of thought and joy untroubled. Do not trouble their joy, don't harass them, don't deprive them of their happiness, don't work against God's intent. Man, do not pride yourself on superiority to animals; they are without sin, and you, with your greatness, defile the earth by your appearance on it, and leave the traces of your foulness after you—alas, it is true of almost every one of us!"

Rabbi David Rosen, Author of "Vegetarianism: An Orthodox Jewish Perspective" in *Rabbis and Vegetarianism: An Evolving Tradition* (1995)

The current treatment of animals in the livestock trade definitely renders the consumption of meat as halachically unacceptable as the product of illegitimate means… As it is halachically prohibited to harm oneself and as healthy, nutritious vegetarian alternatives are easily available, meat consumption has become halachically unjustifiable.

Dr. Albert Schweitzer (1875–1965), physician, missionary, theologian, and Nobel Prize winner

"Until he extends the circle of his compassion to all living things, man will not himself find peace."

"Let no one regard as light the burden of his responsibility. While so much ill-treatment of animals goes on, while the moans of thirsty animals in railway trucks sound unheard, while so much brutality prevails in our slaughterhouses…we all bear guilt. Everything that lives has value as a living thing, as one of the manifestations of the mystery that is life. It is the fate of every truth to be an object of ridicule when it is first acclaimed. It was once considered foolish to suppose that black men were really human beings and ought to be treated as such. What was once foolish has now become a recognized truth. Today it is considered as exaggeration to proclaim constant respect for every form of life as being the serious demand of a rational ethic. But the time is coming when people will be amazed that the human race existed so long before it recognized that thoughtless injury to life is incompatible with real ethics. Ethics is in its unqualified form extended responsibility to everything that has life."

"The thinking man must oppose all cruel customs no matter how deeply rooted in tradition and surrounded by a halo. When we have a choice, we must avoid bringing torment and injury into the life of another, even the lowliest creature; to do so is to renounce our manhood and shoulder a guilt which nothing justifies."

Dr. Walter Willett, Chair of the Department of Nutrition, Harvard University

"If you step back and look at the data, the optimum amount of red meat you eat should be zero."

Thomas Edison (1847–1931), fourth most prolific inventor in history

"Nonviolence leads to the highest ethics, which is the goal of all evolution. Until we stop harming all other living beings, we are still savages."

Charles Darwin (1809–1882), author of *On the Origin of Species*

"The love for all living creatures is the most noble attribute of man."

Rev. John Dear, Jesuit priest, peace activist, author of twenty books on Christian discipleship, and former head of the Fellowship of Reconciliation

"A vegetarian diet is the only diet for people who care about the suffering of other people. Domestically, slaughterhouses are dens of death not just for animals, but for the unfortunate people who work in them. Slaughterhouses have the highest rate of injury, the highest turnover rate, the highest repeat-injury rate, and the highest rate of accidental death of any industry in the country."

Robert Louis Stevenson (1850–1894), Scottish novelist among whose works are *Treasure Island* and *The Strange Case of Dr. Jekyll and Mr. Hyde*

"We consume the carcasses of creatures of like appetites, passions and organs as our own, and fill the slaughterhouses daily with screams of pain and fear."

Dr. Neal Barnard, President of the Physicians Committee for Responsible Medicine and Professor, George Washington University Medical School

"The beef industry has contributed to more American deaths than all the wars of this century, all natural disasters, and all automobile accidents combined. If beef is your idea of 'real food for real people,' you'd better live real close to a real good hospital."

Rabbi Moses ben Maino (1135–1204), Jewish theologian and codifier of the Talmud

"It should not be believed that all beings exist for the sake of the existence of man. On the contrary, all the other beings too have been intended for their own sakes and not for the sake of anything else."

"[Regarding animals and their offspring], there is no difference between the pain of humans and the pain of other living beings, since the love and tenderness of the mother for the young are not produced by reasoning, but by feeling, and this faculty exists not only in humans but in most living beings."

Immanuel Kant (1724–1804), world-renowned German philosopher

"We can judge the heart of a man by his treatment of animals."

Sir Arthur Conan Doyle (1859–1930), Scottish physician, author, and novelist best known for his fictional stories about the detective Sherlock Holmes

"At the moment our human world is based on the suffering and destruction of millions of nonhumans. To perceive this and to do something to change it in personal and public ways is to undergo a change of perception akin to a religious conversion. Nothing can ever be seen in quite the same way again because once you have admitted the terror and pain of other species you will, unless you resist conversion, be always aware of the endless permutations of suffering that support our society."

Voltaire (1694–1778), French Enlightenment philosopher and writer known for his advocacy of personal liberties and separation of church and state

"People must have renounced, it seems to me, all natural intelligence to dare to advance that animals are but animated machines...It appears to me, besides, that [such people] can never have observed with attention the character of animals, not to have distinguished among them the different voices of need, of suffering, of joy, of pain, of love, of anger, and of all their affections. It would be very strange that they should express so well what they could not feel."

"How pitiful, and what poverty of mind, to have said that the animals are machines deprived of understanding and feeling. Judge (in the same way as you would judge your own) the behaviour of a dog who has lost his master, who has searched for him in the road barking miserably, who has come back to the house restless and anxious, who has run upstairs and down, from room to room, and who has found the beloved master at last in his study, and then shown his joy by barks, bounds and caresses. There are some barbarians who will take this dog, that so greatly excels man in capacity for friendship, who will nail him to a table, and dissect him alive, in order to show you his veins and nerves. And what you then discover in him are all the same organs of sensation that you have in yourself. Answer me, mechanist, has Nature arranged all the springs of feeling in this animal to the end that he might not feel? Has he nerves that he may be incapable of suffering?"

The Prophet Mohammed (570–632), Islamic prophet who unified Arabia into a single religious polity under Islam

"A good deed done to an animal is as meritorious as a good deed done to a human being, while an act of cruelty to an animal is as bad as an act of cruelty to a human being."

Sir Paul McCartney, iconic songwriter, singer, and musician

"If slaughterhouses had glass walls, the whole world would be vegetarian."

Henry David Thoreau (1817–1862), author and naturalist best known for his book *Walden*, a reflection upon simple living in natural surroundings

"No humane being, past the thoughtless age of boyhood, will wantonly murder any creature which holds its life by the same tenure that he does."

Ruth Harrison (1920–2000), Quaker, animal welfare activist, recipient of the chivalry Order of the British Empire, and author of *Animal Machines*

"In fact, if one person is unkind to an animal it is considered to be cruelty, but where a lot of people are unkind to animals, especially in the name of commerce, the cruelty is condoned and, once large sums of money are at stake, will be defended to the last by otherwise intelligent people."

Dr. Colin Campbell, Professor Emeritus of Nutritional Biochemistry, Cornell University, and Senior Science Advisor to the American Institute for Cancer Research

"What we have come to consider as 'normal' illnesses of aging are really not normal. In fact, these findings indicate that the vast majority, perhaps 80 to 90 percent of all cancers, cardiovascular diseases, and other forms of degenerative illness can be prevented, at least until very old age, simply by adopting a plant-based diet. In the next ten to fifteen years, one of the things you're bound to hear is that animal protein is one of the most toxic nutrients of all that can be considered. Risk for disease goes up dramatically when even a little animal protein is added to the diet. We are basically a vegetarian species and should be eating a wide variety of plant food and minimizing our intake of animal foods."

Mohandas Gandhi (1869–1948), Hindu advocate of nonviolent civil disobedience and leading figure of Indian nationalism and self-rule

"I hold that the more helpless a creature, the more entitled it is to protection by man from the cruelty of man."

William Ralph Inge (1860–1954), Professor of Divinity at Cambridge and Dean of St. Paul's Cathedral

"We have enslaved the rest of the animal creation, and have treated our distant cousins in fur and feathers so badly that beyond doubt, if they were able to formulate a religion, they would depict the Devil in human form."

Dr. Elliot Katz, DVM and founder of In Defense of Animals

"The rights of animals are birthrights, similar to those we claim for ourselves—the right to live our lives free of subjugation and institutionalized violence, where the random and special joys of being alive can be experienced."

Russell Simmons, music promoter and cofounder of the hip-hop label Def Jam

"I was raised eating meat just like most other Americans. I believed that finishing my dinner and gulping down my milk would make me grow up to be big and strong...Never once did I consider exactly what I was eating or what happened to the animal before it reached my plate."

Alicia Silverstone, actress, model, and author

"Like most people, I wasn't always a vegetarian, but I've always loved animals. If you ever have a chance to meet a cow, pig, turkey, or goat, you will see that they are just as cute and funny as your dogs and cats and that they, too, want to live and feel love. They don't like pain. Now when I see a steak, it makes me feel sad and sick because right away, I see my dog or the amazing cows I met at a sanctuary."

Gautama Buddha (c.563–483 BC), spiritual philosopher whose teaching became the foundation of Buddhism

"It is more important to prevent animal suffering, rather than sit to contemplate the evils of the universe praying in the company of priests."

Cardinal John Henry Newman (1801–1890), Anglican priest who converted to Roman Catholicism and leader of the Anglican Oxford Movement who was beatified by Pope Benedict XVI in 2010

"Cruelty to animals is as if man did not love God."

"Now what is it moves our very heart and sickens us so much as cruelty shown to poor brutes? I suppose this: first, that they have done us no harm; next, that they have no power whatever of resistance; it is the cowardice and tyranny of which they are the victims which make their sufferings so especially touching."

"There is something so dreadful, so Satanic, in tormenting those who have never harmed us, and who cannot defend themselves, who are utterly in our power."

John Ray (1628–1704), British naturalist and developer of the botanical classification system

"There is no doubt, that man is not built to be a carnivorous animal...What a sweet, pleasing and innocent sight is the spectacle of a table served that way and what a difference to a make up of fuming animal meat, slaughtered and dead! Man in no way has the constitution of a carnivorous being. Hunt and voracity are unnatural to him. Man has neither the sharp pointed teeth or claws to slaughter his prey. On the contrary his hands are made to pick fruits, berries and vegetables and teeth appropriate to chew them…Everything we need to feed ourselves and to restore and please us is abundantly provided in the inexhaustible store of Nature. In short our orchards offer all the delights imaginable while the slaughter houses and butchers are full of congealed blood and abominable stench."

Dr. Caldwell Esselstyn, former President of the Staff and member of the Board of Governors of the Cleveland Clinic and author of the landmark book *Prevent and Reverse Heart Disease*, which documented his twelve-year clinical trial with heart patients demonstrating that a whole-grains-plant–based diet can halt and even reverse coronary artery disease

"Here are the facts. Coronary artery disease is the leading killer of men and women in Western civilization. In the United States alone, more than half a million people die of it every single year. Three times that number suffer known heart attacks. And approximately three million more have 'silent' heart attacks, experiencing minimal symptoms and having no idea, until well after the damage is done, that they are in mortal danger. In the course of a lifetime, one out of every two American men and one out of every three American women will have some form of the disease.

"Every mouthful of oils and animal products, including dairy foods, initiates an assault on these [cell] membranes and, therefore, on the cells they protect. These foods produce a cascade of free radicals in our bodies—especially harmful chemical substances that induce metabolic injuries from which there is only a partial recovery. Year after year, the effects accumulate. And eventually, the cumulative cell injury is great enough to become obvious, to express itself as what physicians define as disease."

"Plants and grains do not induce the deadly cascade of free radicals. Even better, in fact, they carry an antidote. Unlike oils and animal products, they contain antioxidants, which help to neutralize the free radicals and also, recent research suggests, may provide considerable protection against cancers."

George Bernard Shaw (1856–1950), playwright of over sixty plays, winner of the 1925 Nobel Prize in Literature, and cofounder of the London School of Economics

"While we ourselves are the living graves of murdered beasts, how can we expect any ideal conditions on this earth? Animals are my friends...and I don't eat my friends."

Think about that succinct yet profound last statement, "Animals are my friends. I don't eat my friends." Do you consider yourself a friend to animals? Isn't that reason enough to never let another morsel of animal flesh pass your lips?

These quotes are from so many people, from so many walks of life, spanning so many centuries, each independently speaking out about the benefits of not eating the animals. Yet most of us do not listen.

Consequently, the suffering goes on. Millions of animals live miserable, unnatural lives and die gruesome premature deaths. Slaughterhouse workers continue to endure psychic damage and bodily injury. Our environment absorbs tons more unnecessary pollutants, and limited arable land that could be used to grow food for the hungry poor continues to be depleted to raise animals for the wealthy. All of this is while our arteries clog with plaque and we suffer avoidable strokes, heart attacks, and certain cancers that kill us and rob our families of our presence far earlier than God or nature ever intended.

At what point does a rational person with a compassionate heart stop ignoring the facts and embrace the life-affirming wisdom that comes to us through the ages?

Stop eating the animals.

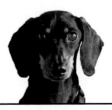

If you love your pets at home, please liberate
their imprisoned cousins on the factory farms
by adopting a healthy meat-free foodstyle.

7
A POSITIVE PERSONAL CHOICE

Frances Moore Lappe, author of the ground-breaking book *Diet for a Small Planet,* wisely said "Every aspect of our lives is, in a sense, a vote for the kind of world we want to live in." She's right. Each of us is a free moral agent who can choose most aspects of how we live our lives. Nowhere are those choices so open than in the developed world, where we have such an abundance of resources available to us. This affords us the opportunity to ask ourselves, do we want our food choices to needlessly continue a cycle of violence against innocent animals? Or do we want to promote the health and well-being of ourselves, our families, and other people as well the animals with whom we share this planet?

We are all familiar with the ethical precept about reciprocity known as "The Golden Rule." It says that we should treat others as we'd like to be treated. And that we should not do to others what we wouldn't want done to us. Most of us would neither bite a dog nor want to be bitten, or deny a cat her daily meals any more than we'd want to be denied ours. We wouldn't imprison a cow for most of her life any more than we'd want to be imprisoned during our life. Most of us wouldn't want to be trapped, confined, and killed in order to have our skin peeled off our bodies so someone else can wear it as fashion. Most women wouldn't take a calf away from her mother any more than she'd want her children taken away from her. No man would volunteer to have his genitals ripped off his body as many male pigs have done to them. None of us would want any of these things done to us. Yet the truth is, each time we heat up a meatloaf, cook a ham, or grill a chicken, we promote the very activities that we would not want done to us.

The Universal Appeal of the Golden Rule

CHRISTIANITY	"In everything, do to others as you would have them do to you; for this is the law and the prophets." *Jesus, Gospel of Matthew 7:12*
JUDAISM	"What is hateful to you, do not do to your neighbor. This is the whole Torah; all the rest is commentary." *Hillel, Talmud, Shabbat 31a*
ISLAM	"Not one of you truly believes until you wish for others what you wish for yourself." *The Prophet Muhammad, Hadith*
HINDUISM	"This is the sum of duty: do not do to others what would cause pain if done to you." *Mahabharata 5:1517*

BUDDHISM	"Treat not others in ways that you yourself would find hurtful." *Udana-Varga 5:18*
SIKHISM	"I am a stranger to no one; and no one is a stranger to me. Indeed, I am a friend to all." *Guru Granth Sahib, pg. 1299*
TAOSIM	"Regard your neighbor's gain as your own gain, and your neighbor's loss as your own loss." *T'ai Shang Kan Ying P'ien, 213–218*
CONFUCIANISM	"One word which sums up the basis of all good conduct...loving kindness. Do not do to others what you do not want done to yourself." *Confucious, Analects 15.23*
ZOROASTRIANISM	"Do not do unto others whatever is injurious to yourself."*Shayast-na-Shayast 13.29*
BAHA'I FAITH	"Lay not on any soul a load that you would not wish to be laid upon you, and desire not for anyone the things you would not desire for yourself." *Baha'ullah, Gleanings*
NATIVE SPIRITUALITY	"We are as much alive as we keep the earth alive." *Chief Dan George*

| JAINISM | "One should treat all creatures in the world as one would like to be treated." *Mahavina, Sutrakritanga* |

If we are to be true to ourselves, to those values to which we say we subscribe, to those actions that we hope our children will emulate, we cannot continue to treat animals with cruelty, callousness, or ambivalence. Only a hypocrite treats others miserably and then complains when others treat him the same way. The ethic of reciprocity is universal and timeless.

Much as we may covet the flesh, feather, or fur of animals, it is not ours to take. It belongs to them. It is their muscles that animate their bodies. It is their covering that keeps them cool and clean. It is their coats that keep them warm through the cold winter. All animals have a right to their bodies. They know how to enjoy their lives and, unless they are attacking us or we are starving, we have no right to deprive them of life or limb.

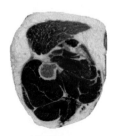 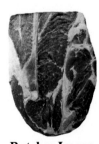

NIH Image **Butcher Image**

Consider these two cross-sectional images of musculature, cartilage, fat, and bone. While they look similar and would probably respond comparably to the application of high heat on a grill, it's worth noting that the image on the right is from a cow, while the one on the left is from a human. Animals' bodies feel and function just as ours do. Animals live, breathe, and move in space and time just as we do. Animals seek self-preservation no less than we do. Shouldn't they, like us, be able to live their lives as God and nature intended? They don't want to be eaten any more than we do.

Within the 46 percent of American households with dogs and 39 percent with cats live mostly kind-hearted people who have made a connection with special animals, the canine and feline "Ambassadors of the Animal Kingdom." We come to understand that these creatures are every bit as interested in their lives as we are in our own through their relationships of care and affection; in observing their habits and happiness; in developing routines of daily life and activities together; in being amused at their antics and touched by their cuteness; in empathizing with their hunger, loneliness, sickness, and aging; and in feeling their presence and loss. They teach us that, though each species may have its own unique anatomy, physiology, language, and behaviors, what they and we share in common is the breath of life given to us by the same source. We are the handiwork of the same creator and are made of the same matter, and our bodies have the same temporal destiny. It is true of dog and duck, cat and cow, eagle and elephant, pig and possum, horse and, yes, human.

Remember what is written in Ecclesiastes: *"For what happens to the children of man and what happens to the beasts is the same; as one dies, so dies the other. They all have the same breath, and man has no advantage*

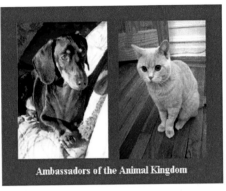

Ambassadors of the Animal Kingdom

over the beasts, for all is vanity. All go to one place. All are from the dust, and to dust all return."

God in His eternal wisdom has granted to us humans made in His image, and to the creatures whom He has entrusted to our care, feeling bodies through which we sojourn on this earth. His animals travel with us. If we don't accord them the same consideration, irrespective of species, then we're not paying adequate attention to what the ambassadors from the animal kingdom are trying to teach us—that all animals love their lives and deserve to live out their natural lives free of destructive human interference.

Consider why cows are consumed aplenty in America but are sacred in India, or why dogs are eaten in some Asian countries but are doted upon in the West. It is not because of any existential differences but merely due to cultural prerogatives. And even within a single culture the messages are often conflicting. Bambi is a beloved childhood fable character, yet deer are shot in the woods for sport. Donald Duck elicits laughter from our kids, yet on factory farms ducks are force-fed to grotesque proportions to enlarge their livers for us to eat. Porky Pig is an engaging cartoon character, yet pigs are imprisoned and brutalized daily. The childrens' fables are few, but the tales of real animal suffering are endless.

We are the adults. We know the difference between fantasy and reality. The reality is that no animal wants to be imprisoned and eaten by another creature. It suffices in the wild where nature dictates who lives and who dies. But in civilized societies of abundance such as our own, rational minds and compassionate hearts can protest senseless suffering and slaughter. We can make positive personal choices, and that can begin by making a commitment to ourselves that the flesh of animals shall no longer pass our lips.

How we may come to make that choice will differ for each person. Some may be motivated to improve their own and their families' health, perhaps to lower cholesterol levels, reduce cancer risk, or lose weight. Others may be motivated by compassion for the suffering of the animals. Still others may be prompted by a desire to see more agricultural land devoted to raising plants to feed the world's poor, to spare low-wage workers the psychic damage of laboring in slaughterhouses, or to reduce the harmful impact of factory farming on our environment.

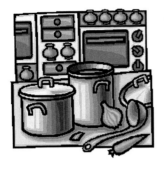

Whatever the motivation, choosing to stop eating the animals could be one of your life's most noble actions of which you can be rightly proud. You will feel more empowered, empathetic, and energized. And you will enjoy it. It's hard not to. You will physically feel better. You will emotionally feel more at peace and connected to all living creatures. And you will spiritually grow in awareness of your authentic self as a more caring, thoughtful, and peaceful person who eschews violence wherever it's found—even in our kitchens.

Making such a decision will represent a big change and, with change, also comes uncertainty. That is normal and to be expected. In this case, the discomfort of change will be short lived and will ultimately prove interesting, beneficial, and even fun. You will be embarking upon a journey and discovering culinary choices that are tasty, satisfying, and healthy, while making a contribution to animal welfare, world hunger, our environment, and your own health.

For those who elect to take that journey, I wish you bon voyage!

If all creatures praise God, humans should not be killing some of the choir members!

8

TRANSITIONING TO A MEAT-FREE FOODSTYLE

So you're interested in eliminating animal flesh from your diet. What do you eat? What do you buy? What do you cook? Adopting a diet without animal flesh is easier than you may think. Many folks who were meat eaters for much of their lives have transitioned and never looked back because the food can be equally delicious, and they've learned to use food to enhance, rather than harm, their health.

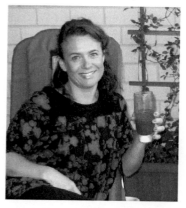

Perhaps most convincing is that they feel better. They have more energy throughout the day, feel mentally more alert and clearer in their thinking, no longer feel lethargic after eating, often drop excess pounds, and live free of worrying that the food they put into their mouths is diminishing their health. The transition isn't so much a dietary change as much as the adoption of a *'foodstyle'* premised upon a paradigm shift in thinking to be an advocate for your own and your family's health, while advancing the well-being of innocent animals and reducing pollution. Actions borne of this thinking engender an internal feeling of peace.

Humans are amazingly adaptable. Like most things to which we've become accustomed, foods can also be changed with no sense of deprivation. Many people report that it takes about two to four weeks for their palates to adjust to eating meat-free meals. This foodstyle is based upon a diet comprised of vegetables, legumes, grains, fruits, nuts, and seeds. There are several variations, which can get a bit confusing, but they all essentially derive from the Latin word *vegetus*, which means full of vitality and vigor.

Some dictionaries define *vegetarianism* as only avoiding the consumption of mammal flesh as meat, but allowing consumption of fish, while others extend the definition of vegetarianism to exclude fish and seafood as well as the meat of mammals. It is worth being aware of the several variations of the meat-free foodstyle.

Vegetarians are generally considered to not consume the flesh of any animals. Some also avoid products containing animal ingredients, such as the enzymes from animals' stomach lining called *rennet* that is used in the production of certain cheeses, sugars whitened with bone char, and gelatin derived from the collagen in animals' skin and connective tissue. Often these ingredients are not listed on product labels, so it is difficult to ascertain whether a product contains them or not. *Vegans* avoid eating all animal flesh as well as all animal products, such as dairy and honey. Some also avoid nonedible animal products such as leather, fur, and feathers. *Raw vegans* avoid animal products and limit themselves to uncooked or minimally cooked vegetables, fruits, and nuts. *Semivegetarians* are less restrictive in what they won't eat. *Pescetarians* avoid the flesh of mammals but may eat fish and seafood. *Lacto-vegetarians* avoid animal flesh and eggs but will eat diary products. *Ovo-vegetarians* won't eat animal flesh or dairy but will eat eggs. *Ovo-lacto-vegetarians* avoid animal flesh but will eat eggs, dairy, and honey.

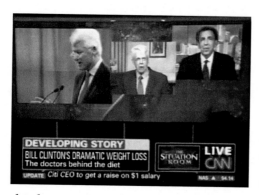

More recently an additional category of the meat-free foodstyle has emerged to address specific health needs. Based largely upon the recommendations of such pioneering thinkers as Drs. Caldwell Esselstyn, Dean Ornish, and T. Colin Campbell, it's known as a *whole grains, plant-based diet*. It essentially posits that the healthiest diet is one that avoids eating anything "with a mother or a face." That includes mammals as well as fish. It also prohibits or limits the intake of eggs, dairy, and certain oils and fats. Their independent research and clinical trials have revealed that animal protein can inflame our artery walls and trigger cancer cell growth. With heart disease in particular, this diet can stop and reverse arteriosclerosis. This is the life-saving diet that former President Bill Clinton adopted a few years ago. You may wish to go online to see CNN's "Situation Room" interview of President Clinton along with Drs. Esselstyn and Ornish.

You will recall that the American Dietetic Association advised that "Well-planned vegetarian diets are appropriate for individuals during all stages of the life cycle, including, pregnancy, lactation, infancy, childhood, and adolescence, and for athletes." But how do you know if you are getting all the nutrients that you need if you give up animal sources of protein? The Mayo Clinic, the first and largest integrated nonprofit medical group practice in the world, celebrating 150 years of continuous service to patients in 2014, provides sound advice worth considering.

Mayo Clinic

Getting Adequate Nutrition

The key to a healthy vegetarian diet—like any diet—is to enjoy a variety of foods. No single food can provide all the nutrients your body needs. The more restrictive your diet is, the more challenging it can be to get all the the nutrients you need. A vegan diet, for example, eliminates natural food sources of vitamin B-12, as well as milk products, which are good sources of calcium. With a little planning, however, you can be sure that your diet includes everything your body needs. Pay special attention to the following nutrients:

Calcium helps build and maintain strong teeth and bones. Milk and dairy foods are highest in calcium. However, dark green vegetables, such as turnip and collard greens, kale and broccoli, are good plant sources when eaten in sufficient quantities. Calcium-enriched and fortified products, including juices, cereals, soy milk, soy yogurt and tofu, are other options.

Iodine is a component in thyroid hormones, which help regulate metabolism, growth and function of key organs. Vegans may not get enough iodine and be at risk of deficiency and possibly even a goiter. In addition, foods such as soybeans, cruciferous vegetables and sweet potatoes may promote a goiter. However, just 1/4 teaspoon of iodized salt provides a significant amount of iodine.

Iron is a crucial component of red blood cells. Dried beans and peas, lentils, enriched cereals, whole-grain products, dark leafy green vegetables and dried fruit are good sources of iron. Because iron isn't as easily absorbed from plant sources, the recommended intake of iron for vegetarians is almost double that recommended for nonvegetarians. To help your body absorb iron, eat foods rich in vitamin C, such as strawberries, citrus fruits, tomatoes, cabbage and broccoli, at the same time as you're eating iron-containing foods.

Omega-3 fatty acids are important for heart health. Diets that do not include fish and eggs are generally low in active forms of omega-3 fatty acids. Canola oil, soy oil, walnuts, ground flaxseed and soybeans are good sources of essential fatty acids. However, because conversion of plant-based omega-3 to the types used by humans is inefficient, you may want to consider fortified products or supplements, or both.

Protein helps maintain healthy skin, bones, muscles and organs. Eggs and dairy products are good sources, and you don't need to eat large amounts to meet your protein needs. You can also get sufficient protein from plant-based foods if you eat a variety of them throughout the day. Plant sources include soy products and meat substitutes, legumes, lentils, nuts, seeds and whole grains.

Vitamin B-12 is necessary to produce red blood cells and prevent anemia. This vitamin is found almost exclusively in animal products, so it can be difficult to get enough B-12 on a vegan diet. Vitamin B-12 deficiency may go undetected in people who eat a vegan diet. This is because the vegan diet is rich in a vitamin called folate, which may mask deficiency in vitamin B-12 until severe problems occur. For this reason, it's important for vegans to consider vitamin supplements, vitamin-enriched cereals and fortified soy products.

Vitamin D plays an important role in bone health. Vitamin D is added to cow's milk, some brands of soy and rice milk, and some cereals and margarines. Be sure to check food labels. If you don't eat enough fortified foods and have limited sun exposure, you may need a vitamin D supplement (one derived from plants).

Zinc is an essential component of many enzymes and plays a role in cell division and in formation of proteins. Like iron, zinc is not as easily absorbed from plant sources as it is from animal products. Cheese is a good option if you eat dairy products. Plant sources of zinc include whole grains, soy products, legumes, nuts and wheat germ.

If you need help creating a vegetarian diet that's right for you, talk with your doctor and a registered dietitian.

© Mayo Clinic

Variations of vegan, vegetarian, pescetarian, plant-based, and other diets can be confusing. Some folks may still occasionally eat fish and seafood, particularly when first beginning this new way of thinking about food, but what people who have adopted basic meat-free foodstyles share in common is they stopped eating land mammals, marine mammals, and birds. One can imagine to the relief of many animals who would otherwise end up on someone's dinner plate, including antelope, bears, beavers, bison, boars, bobcats, buffalo, camels, chickens, cows, coyotes, deer, dolphins, doves, ducks, elephants, elk, emus, geese, goats, guinea fowl, kangaroos, lambs, lions, llamas, manatees, monkeys, moose, muskrat, opossums, ostrich, otters, partridge, peacocks, pheasants, pigeons, pigs, porpoises, quail, rabbits, reindeer, sea lions, sheep, turkeys, walruses, water buffalo, whales, yaks, zebras, and others.

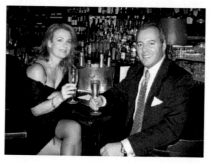

When my wife and I decided to adopt a meat-free foodstyle, we made two commitments to ourselves. First, we agreed that we would not allow ourselves to feel deprived, because if we did, we would not stick with the change. No one wants to feel deprived. That is not an effective motivator. So to ensure that we did not feel any sense of deprivation, we decided to go meat-free six days a week and allow ourselves one day a week—Sundays or holidays—to eat and drink whatever we wished.

But an interesting thing happened on our way to a restaurant that first Sunday. Once we made that paradigm shift in thinking, even though we gave ourselves the freedom to eat anything that day, when we sat down at our favorite brunch restaurant and looked at the menu, we were more drawn to meatless dishes. We no longer wanted meat. Desire for healthier food had trumped any sense of deprivation. We felt liberated!

Knowing that we could have meat if we wanted it eliminated any sense of sacrifice or loss. We were free to eat whatever we wished. We chose to eat meat-free appetizers and entrees and thoroughly enjoyed them as much as we had previously enjoyed meat-based meals. It helped that we adopted a healthy mental posture to encourage healthy actions. Instead of feeling as if we might miss something, we felt that we dodged an artery-clogging bullet and gained a measure of better health.

Second, we agreed that our meat-free meals would have to taste good. We were both accustomed to eating finely prepared foods, rich in flavor and variety, thanks in part to my wife's creativity in the kitchen as well as to our living in New York City, with its plethora of restaurants serving delicious cuisines from all over the world. Moreover, earlier in our careers before we met, my wife and I each had corporate expense accounts and entertained clients at some of the best restaurants. It would be a lie if we said that we hadn't enjoyed eating meat dishes prepared by some of the city's finest chefs. We certainly did. But much as we enjoyed eating that way then, today we can't even bear to walk by the refrigerated meat section of the supermarket without seeing not steaks, sausages, and sirloin but dead animal body parts. It saddens us and was one of the motivations for me to write this book.

Even though we no longer eat meat, our desire for tasty food has not abated. We won't settle for bland, boring food either at home or in a restaurant. Like most people, we like our food to have a pleasing taste and texture. How we have come to enjoy our food just as much as before has a lot to do with creativity in the kitchen, experimenting with new foods, plentiful use of herbs, and clever application of exotic spices. The result is that we have experienced previously unknown flavors, learned about once-overlooked nutritional content, and enhanced our energy levels and overall health.

Not every meal, of course, is a carefully crafted creation. We have neither the time nor the inclination for that every day. Most meals, in fact, are easily prepared dishes of foods that we know and relish that can be put on the table quickly after a long day at work. Some days we just like to eat comfort foods, the meatless ones that we know are healthy.

> "The secret of change is to focus all of your energy, not on fighting the old, but on building the new."
>
> Socrates (470–399 BC)

One potential obstacle that you may experience in making the transition is psychological. You may be so conditioned to seeing meat in some shape or form on your plate that you may think that something is missing. Yes, the animal flesh will be gone, but none of the nutrients since they will be more than adequately provided by an assortment of vegetables, legumes, fruits, grains, nuts, and seeds, all of which you can serve in appetizing ways. Your dinner table need never appear bare when you're serving a cornucopia of healthy fare.

In the last several years, as the benefits of avoiding animal flesh have emerged from research and clinical studies, the market has been filling with recipes and cookbooks to help people make the transition to healthier eating without meat. The more you learn about the toll that eating animal flesh takes on our bodies, and the benefits of eating more plants and grains, the easier it will be for you to stick with this change. Go online and do some research. You'll be amazed at how many people are coming around to a meat-free foodstyle.

It's still in the relatively early stages, but the trend is unmistakable. You see it in the growing number of vegetarian and vegan restaurants, grocery stores devoted to organic foods, and nonanimal foods stocked on traditional supermarket shelves.

Here are a few resources that we found helpful when starting our transition to a meat-free foodstyle"

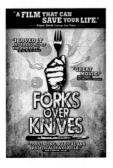

Forks Over Knives is available as a DVD or a book. The DVD can form the basis of a movie night with friends to share emerging health information that can literally save lives.

Prevent and Reverse Heart Disease reports on the clinical study conducted by Dr. Caldwell Esselstyn on patients whose heart disease was not only arrested but in some cases actually reversed through diet alone.

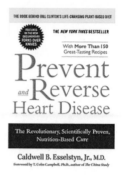

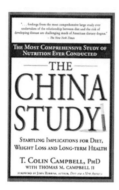

The China Study by T. Colin Campbell and Thomas M. Campbell describes the connections between nutrition and heart disease, diabetes, and cancer and has been hailed as the most comprehensive large study ever undertaken of the relationship between diet and the risk of developing disease.

Dr. Dean Ornish is the first clinician to document that heart disease can be halted or even reversed by changing one's lifestyle. His "Opening Your Heart Program" goes beyond the purely physical aspect of health to include the psychological, emotional, and spiritual. Participants in his study reduced or discontinued medications, lost weight, and reduced coronary artery blockages. He is primarily credited with helping former

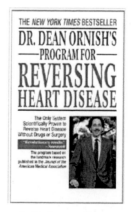

President Clinton deal with his life-threatening cardiovascular problems.

Among the many good cookbooks on the market, my wife found these two very helpful— *Forks Over Knives The Cookbook* by Del Sroufe with desserts by Isa 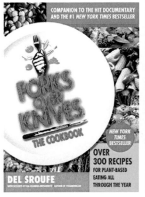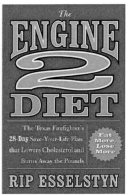 Chandra Moskowitz, and *The Engine 2 Diet* by Rip Esselstyn. You'll be surprised at how many overlooked vegetables are just bursting with flavor and nutrition, and perhaps even more amazed at the types of food combinations that will be as palate-pleasing as any meal you have ever served your family.

Before my wife and I even delved into the cookbooks, however, we decided to go to a few popular vegetarian and vegan restaurants to see what good plant-based fare looked and tasted like. We were not disappointed.

The first venue that we chose had the look, feel, and even the prices of the other fine restaurants that we used to frequent. This particular one had wood paneling, elegant lighting, plush seating, a smartly fashioned bar attended by beautiful people, an extensive wine list, and a menu that stimulated our imaginations as much as our taste buds.

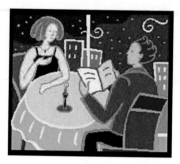

Our first reaction that night was relief! We were thrilled that, in order to adopt this meat-free foodstyle, we wouldn't have to survive on rabbit food or eat in spartan surroundings. We could enjoy the same lifestyle to which we had become accustomed while embracing a meat-free foodstyle. Needless to say, we ordered several different dishes that night and marveled at how good they were. Some items we had never even heard of before, but they were so tasty that we were determined to learn their ingredients and look for them at the grocery store. Even their beverage list caused a flight of fancy. Who knew that fruits and vegetables could be composed into cocktails of such splendid taste and sophistication?

That night inspired us to try several other vegetarian and vegan restaurants, not all high brow. In fact, most of them were far more modest venues, but the quality of food coming out of their kitchens was no less impressive. We were convinced. Adopting a meat-free foodstyle composed of vegetables, legumes, grains, fruits, nuts, and seeds does not require sacrifice and does not create a feeling of deprivation. Quite the contrary. Once you learn your way around the vegetarian and vegan menu and bring these foods into your home, eating this way adds a new, interesting, and enjoyable dimension to your life. You can look forward to new culinary experiences and shed guilt and pounds in the process. Adopting a meat-free food-style brings an abundance of marvelous fun as well as healthy food!

During the initial transition period, you may experience an aversion to meat with a concomitant desire for fresh foods. Welcome that awareness as an important telltale sign that your mind, as well as your body, is adapting to this healthy meat-free foodstyle.

While you are testing your palates by eating at some vegetarian and vegan restaurants, ask questions of your wait staff. Most of them will be quite happy to share information with you because they are more often than not already committed to a meat-free foodstyle themselves. They can guide you to selections that you'll most likely enjoy and can explain the ingredients that go into each dish. Be discrete but take notes. You'll want to shop for some of the ingredients that they mention so that you can prepare similar dishes at home. And don't skip the desserts. My wife and I have been introduced to some veg desserts that would be the envy of any pastry chef!

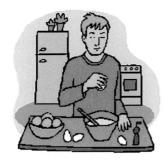

After you've had your fill of restaurant fare and realize that this type of food can be just as delicious as what you used to eat, it's time to open some cookbooks. In them you will find plenty of healthy dishes that you can make at home. Don't overwhelm yourself. Just pick a few, note their ingredients, and go shopping with the idea of making one or two special meals. Then have fun and experiment.

Realistically, you should be prepared to make a few meals that don't impress. It's inevitable in any creative process. No one hits a home run every time at bat. In our experience, we decided that 10 percent of the meals my wife prepared were "first and last time." They just didn't taste good. Perfectly healthy but just not flavorful enough to eat again. Another 70 percent were very tasty, sometimes amazingly tasty because of their new ingredients, and became regular fare in our home. And then there was the 20 percent that we called my wife's "signature dishes"—meals so delectable that they've become our special holiday dinners.

What we found most intriguing during our initial foray into the meat-free foodstyle was how the delicate flavors of many different vegetables and grains had previously gone unnoticed. Once your palate is free of animal flesh and fat, the nuanced flavors of different grains and vegetables can be more fully appreciated. And thanks to the enhancements of exotic herbs and spices, many carrying their own health benefits, you will be able to stimulate your and your family members' palates with a wide variety of flavors and textures while providing the healthiest forms of nourishment.

So what, you may ask yourself, do I pull out of my refrigerator, put onto my countertop, and prepare as a meal for myself and my family?

The Physicians Committee for Responsible Medicine (PCRM) has a simple graphic to help transition to a plant-based diet. Since its establishment in 1985, the PCRM has been influencing advances in science through its advocacy of preventive medicine, good nutrition, and ethical clinical research. It is led by Dr. Neal Barnard; a Board of Directors that includes Drs. Russell Bunai, Mark Sklar, and Barbara Wasserman; and a highly regarded Advisory Board comprised of leading healthcare practitioners throughout the United States and Canada.

Advisory Board of the Physicians Committee for Responsible Medicine

Leslie Brown, M.D., Pontchartrain Pediatrics

T. Colin Campbell, Ph.D., Cornell University

Caldwell B. Esselstyn, Jr., M.D., The Cleveland Clinic

Roberta Gray, M.D., F.A.A.P., Pediatric Nephrology Consultant

Suzanne Havala Hobbs, Dr.PH., M.S., R.D., University of North Carolina at Chapel Hill

Henry J. Heimlich, M.D., Sc.D., The Heimlich Institute

David Jenkins, M.D., Ph.D., Sc.D., St. Michael's Hospital, Toronto

Lawrence Kushi, Sc.D., Division of Research, Kaiser Permanente

John McDougall, M.D., McDougall Program, St. Helena Hospital

Milton Mills, M.D., Gilead Medical Group

Baxter Montgomery, M.D., Houston Cardiac Association and HCA Wellness Center

Carl Myers, M.D., Sonoran Desert Oncology

Ana Negrón, M.D., Community Volunteers in Medicine and family physician

Myriam Parham, R.D., L.D., C.D.E., East Pasco Medical Center

William Roberts, M.D., Baylor Cardiovascular Institute

Joan Sabaté, M.D., Dr.PH., Loma Linda University Nutrition School of Public Health

Gordon Saxe, M.D., M.P.H., Ph.D., Moores Cancer Center, University of California

Andrew Weil, M.D., University of Arizona

Why The Power Plate?

Plant-Based Diets Promote Health

Science supports a low-fat, plant-based diet for optimal health. The American Dietetic Association (ADA), the nation's largest organization of nutrition experts, states that "vegetarian diets, including total vegetarian or vegan diets, are healthful, nutritionally adequate, and may provide health benefits in the prevention and treatment of certain diseases. Well-planned vegetarian diets are appropriate for individuals during all stages of the lifecycle, including pregnancy, lactation, infancy, childhood, and adolescence, and for athletes."

The ADA's position paper on vegetarian and vegan diets, published in 2009, references more than 200 studies and papers to support its conclusions. Studies continue to show that plant-based diets can aid in reversing the symptoms of America's most devastating diseases: type 2 diabetes, cardiovascular disease, and some types of cancer.

People who follow a plant-based diet have a healthier heart. They reap the benefits of lower cholesterol levels than meat-eaters, and heart disease is less common in vegetarians. Plant-based meals are typically low in saturated fat, and since cholesterol is found only in animal products such as meat, dairy, and eggs, it's easy to consume a cholesterol-free diet.

Another benefit of consuming a plant-based diet is getting your blood pressure numbers down. An impressive number of studies show that vegetarians have lower blood pressure than nonvegetarians. A low-fat, plant-based diet has also shown to reverse the symptoms of type 2 diabetes. A diet based on vegetables, legumes, fruits, and whole grains, which is also low in fat and sugar, can lower blood sugar levels and often reduce or even eliminate the need for medication. Since individuals with diabetes are at high risk for heart disease, avoiding fat and cholesterol is important, and a vegetarian diet is the best way to do that.

A plant-based diet helps prevent cancer. Studies of vegetarians show that death rates from cancer are only about one-half to three-quarters of those of the general population. Breast cancer rates are dramatically lower in countries where diets are typically plant-based.

When people from those countries adopt a Western, meat-based diet, their rates of breast cancer soar. Vegetarians also have significantly lower rates of colon cancer than meat-eaters. Colon cancer is more closely associated with meat consumption than any other dietary factor.

Protective against cancer, plant-based diets are lower in fat and higher in fiber than meat-based diets. They are also full of foods that have phytochemicals, cancer-fighting substances. This might help to explain why vegetarians have less lung and prostate cancer. Also, some studies have suggested that diets that avoid dairy products may reduce the risk of prostate and ovarian cancer.

People who consume plant-based diets are also less likely to form either kidney stones or gallstones. They may also be at lower risk for osteoporosis because they eat little or no animal protein. A high intake of animal protein encourages the loss of calcium from the bones. Replacing animal products with plant foods reduces the amount of calcium lost. This may help to explain why people who live in countries where the diet is typically plant-based have little osteoporosis, even when calcium intake is lower than that in the dairy-consuming countries.

A simple dietary graphic does not replace nutritional teaching, particularly with regard to nutrient adequacy, supplementation, and dietary changes for specific stages of life. It is important to note that vitamin B12 supplementation is essential for individuals following vegan diets. Because of absorption issues, the Dietary Guidelines for Americans and the IOM also recommend vitamin B12 supplementation for all individuals older than 50 years.

Taking control of your quality of life starts with consuming a plant-based diet. Filling your plate with fruits, vegetables, legumes, and grains is not only your best bet for disease prevention, it's an easy way to reverse damage already done. Follow the Power Plate to optimal health.

© Physicians Committee for Responsible Medicine

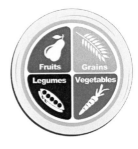

You may wish to learn more about each food group and acquire some recipes by going on PCRM's website at http://pcrm.org/health/diets/pplate/power-plate.

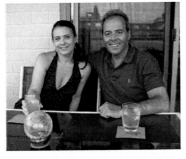

The first month of meals that my wife and I experimented with as novices first making the transition appear in the next chapter. They are real-world examples of what the meat-free foodstyle can look like for breakfast, lunch, and dinner. Although most of the meals were prepared at home, a few were taken at restaurants. Most of those meals my wife has been able to recreate at home, spicing them more precisely for our palates and learning to nutritionally balance them with greater precision.

You'll be pleased to note that these meals take significantly less time to prepare than most animal-based dishes, which require cooking of the meat. Moreover, not having to purchase meat products saves a significant sum of money, making the meat-free foodstyle not only healthier but also more budget friendly. Some of those savings can be used to purchase exotic herbs and spices that will enable the cook in the family to create some remarkably delicious meals, spiced to your own tastes.

Transitioning to the meat-free foodstyle is both challenging and enjoyable at the same time. Have fun with it. Experiment and make your kitchen your adult playroom to develop your own creations. And don't be surprised if you soon find yourself developing a robust appetite for these tasty foods.

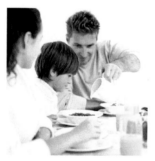

You may want to try foods that you've never experienced before—such as almond milk as a vegan alternative to dairy—and learn how nutritious they are. Experiment with different ingredients, flavors, and textures of food. And remember to serve your meat-free meals with the same casualness or formality that your family is used to so the transition remains in keeping with your traditions at table.

What health benefits can you look forward to if you choose to make the transition to a meat-free foodstyle? A recent article in *The Boston Globe* contained some interesting data that should get the attention of even the most die-hard meat eaters. In her article "Should We Eat Meat?" Karen Weintraub writes, "Although researchers disagree about exactly how much meat is OK to eat, most agree that less is better. Harvard nutrition guru Dr. Walter Willett says he eats red meat only once or twice a year."

She later notes that, "Gary Fraser, who runs a long-range study of 35,000 vegetarians at Loma Linda University in California, said vegetarians fare better than moderate meat-eaters on measures of longevity, heart disease, diabetes, high blood pressure, obesity, and a few cancers. Giving up all animal products, including fish, dairy, and eggs is even better in measures of weight, diabetes, and high blood pressure, his research suggests."

Vegetarians weigh less on average and have a lower risk for diabetes and high blood pressure, which can lead to heart disease, than people who eat meat. Those who eat some chicken and fish and small amounts of red meat have

28%

lower risk of developing diabetes and

23%

lower risk of hypertension than meat-eaters.

Those who eat animal byproducts but no meat have

61%

lower risk of diabetes and

55%

lower risk of hypertension. And vegans have

78%

lower risk of diabetes and

75%

lower risk of hypertension than meat-eaters.

Fish-eaters have

51%

lower risk of diabetes and

38%

lower risk of hypertension than meat-eaters.

© *The Boston Globe*

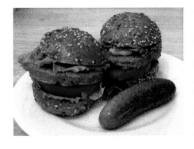

The evidence indicates that the meat-free foodstyle is THE way to nourish ourselves—Tasty, Healthy, and Easy, just like these veggie burgers on multigrain rolls with tomato, shallots, red leaf lettuce, and dijon mustard, served with a garlic barrel pickle. Mmm!

115

9

AN ILLUSTRATIVE FIRST MONTH OF MEALS

Here is a listing of the first thirty-one days of our transitional meat-free meals as novices. While it is not a perfect meal plan, it well served our palate in initially adopting this new foodstyle. Please note that the foods listed are not intended to replace recommendations that you may receive from a physician or nutritionist. You should discuss any dietary changes with your trusted medical professionals, especially if you have any medical conditions, health challenges, or food allergies.

Breakfast	Lunch	Dinner
Fresh fruit salad Ten-grain cereal with rice milk Beverage: tea with lemon and honey	Homemade lentil soup with carrots, onions, parsnip, and whole-wheat round pasta wheels, served with whole-wheat toast Beverage: grape juice with seltzer	Trader Joe's meatless ground beef made of textured wheat and soy protein served warm on endive leaves with bread Fresh garden salad with nonfat dressing Beverage: glass of red wine

Fresh fruit salad of apples, kiwi, and banana Hot steel-cut oatmeal with raisins, flax seed, oat bran, maple syrup, and almond milk	Leftovers of homemade lentil soup with carrots, onions, parsnip, and whole-wheat round pasta wheels, served with Triscuits Beverage: grape juice with seltzer	Trader Joe's meatless ground beef made of textured wheat and soy protein, shredded beets, and Triscuits Green salad with nonfat dressing Beverage: glass of red wine
Fresh apple and red grapes Hot steel-cut oatmeal with maple syrup, raisins, and almond milk Beverage: grape juice with seltzer	Fresh rubbed kale, radicchio, and cucumbers with nonfat dressing, served with whole-wheat toast Beverage: tea	Grilled mushrooms with asparagus and garlic Pasta primavera with tomatoes, peas, zucchini, and broccoli Dessert: chocolate mousse Beverage: glass of red wine and Frangelico
Apple, kiwi, and mandarin orange salad Hot steel-cut oatmeal with flax, raisins, cinnamon, maple syrup, and almond milk Beverage: tea with lemon and honey	Thai sweet and sour soup with garlic, mushrooms, sweet pepper, lime juice, and rice noodles in a vegetable broth Beverage: tea with lemon and honey	Sautéed portobello mushrooms with onions, served with whole-grain barley and steamed broccoli and a side salad of carrots, beets, parsnip, and small white beans Beverage: tea with lemon and honey
Fresh pear and kiwi Oat grains cooked with cinnamon sticks, served with raisins, flax seed,	Mushroom and barley soup with carrots, onions, parsnip, and parsley root, served-with whole-wheat toast	Shredded turnip and celery root with shallots, tossed with lemon soy dressing Salad of chopped cooked parsnip root, beets, carrots, and white beans

maple syrup, and almond milk Beverage: tea with lemon and honey	Beverage: grape juice with seltzer	Mushroom and barley soup served with mini Triscuits Beverage: tea with honey
Fresh pear, kiwi, and red grapes Hot ten-grain cereal with raisins, flax seed, maple syrup, and almond milk Beverage: tea with honey	Tempeh marinated in soy sauce, cooked millet, and mixed vegetables of carrots, beets, parsnip, and white beans Beverage: grape juice with seltzer	Grilled portobello mushroom with onions, served with steamed millet mixed with sautéed onions and black beans Beverage: tea with honey
Fresh apple, kiwi, and red grapes Hot steel-cut oatmeal with flax seed, raisins, maple syrup, and almond milk Beverage: tea with lemon and honey	Tempeh marinated in soy sauce, cooked millet, and steamed spinach with garlic Beverage: tea with honey	Arugula salad with alfalfa sprouts, cucumbers, tomatoes, and shallots tossed with lemon juice and nonfat dressing Mushroom and barley soup with carrots, onions, and parsnip, served with Triscuits Beverage: glass of red wine
Fresh pear, kiwi, and red grapes	Vegetable sushi of mushroom, squash, pickle, asparagus, avocado, and cucumber rolls	Trader Joe's beefless strips made of wheat gluten and isolated soy protein, mixed with Asian stir fry vegetables of peas, broccoli, corn, beans, water chestnuts, and bell pepper in soy sauce, served atop rice noodles

Hot ten-grain cereal with dried cherries, dried blueberries, raisins, flax, maple syrup, and almond milk Beverage: tea with honey	Beverage: ginger ale	Beverage: glass of red wine
Fresh sliced pear Nature's Path organic whole-grain cereal with flax seed, fresh blueberries, and hemp milk Beverage: tea with honey	Leftovers from dinner last night Beverage: grape juice with seltzer	Grilled portobello mushroom served with steamed broccoli with ground pepper and cooked quinoa Beverage: glass of red wine
Bowl of fresh blueberries Hot steel-cut oatmeal with flax seed, raisins, dried cranberries, dried cherries, maple syrup, and hemp milk Beverage: tea with honey	Tri-color salad of wild arugula, radicchio, cucumber, tomato, and shallots, served with a side of tempeh marinated in soyaki sauce Beverage: grape juice with seltzer	Whole-grain pasta shells with grilled portobello mushrooms, fresh tomato, and basil sauce, sprinkled with Parmesan cheese, served with a side of shredded beets spiced with garlic and mesquite Beverage: glass of red wine
Protein shake made with almond milk	Baked potato stuffed with shepherd salad of diced tomatoes, cucumbers, onion,	Baked acorn squash drizzled with maple syrup, served with homemade seventeen bean soup

	and dill, sprinkled with shredded feta cheese Beverage: Turkish tea with sugar	(packaged assortment of beans: baby lima beans, black turtle beans, black-eyed peas, dark red kidney beans, garbanzo beans, great northern beans, green lentils, green split peas, large lima beans, light red kidney beans, wavy beans, pink beans, pinto beans, red lentils, small red beans, small white beans, yellow split peas, and pearl barley), with carrots, celery, chopped onions, parsnip root, and potatos, spiced with smoky paprika chipotle seasoning, celery seed, cumin, bay leaf, and a pinch of Italian seasoning Beverage: dry martini
Fresh fruit salad of pear, red grapes, and banana Hot steel-cut oatmeal with flax seed, raisins, maple syrup, and hemp milk Beverage: grape juice with seltzer	Grilled vegetable sandwich on ciabatta bread with a side of corn and bean salad Beverage: cranberry juice and seltzer	Leftovers from dinner last night, served with Triscuits Beverage: glass of red wine
Fresh pear, apple, and red grapes	Leftover bean and barley soup with Triscuits	Grilled portobello mushroom with steamed

Hot ten-grain cereal with flax seed, raisins, maple syrup, and hemp milk Beverage: water	Snack: Fig Newtons Beverage: grape juice with seltzer	asparagus and quinoa Dessert: oatmeal raisin cookies Beverage: Frangelico
Protein shake made with almond milk	Veggie burger with onions and olives on garlic roll Dessert: oatmeal raisin cookie Beverage: four-fruit juice	Salad of organic arugula, pea shoots, organic baby spinach, cherry tomatoes, shallots, and garlic clove, sprinkled with grated Parmesan cheese and non-fat dressing, served with Triscuits Dessert: piece of 80 percent cocoa dark chocolate Beverage: glass of red wine
Fresh fruit salad Hot ten-grain oatmeal with flax seed, raisins, maple syrup, and hemp milk Beverage: water	Grilled portobello mushroom and onions, served with shredded beets and quinoa Snack: Fig Newton Beverage: grape juice with seltzer	Veggie burger with lettuce and tomato on a roll Beverage: apple juice
Banana Cold cereal made of wheat, oats, barley, millet, and quinoa, with oat bran, raisins, and hemp milk	Trader Joe's chicken-less strips made of isolated soy protein and wheat gluten sautéed in soy sauce with string beans, served with cooked hulled millet mixed with peas and corn	Grilled portobello mushroom, served with Brussels sprouts marinated in soy sauce, red wine, apricot jam, oregano, coriander, and black pepper, and pasta with Parmesan cheese

Beverage: orange juice	Beverage: grape juice with seltzer	Dessert: piece of dark chocolate Beverage: glass of red wine
Fresh pear, kiwi, and red grapes Hot ten-grain cereal with cinnamon, flax seed, raisins, and hemp milk Beverage: grape juice with seltzer	Baked butternut squash mixed with cinnamon and nutmeg, served with tahini and Triscuits Beverage: tea with honey	Vegetarian sushi of cucumber, squash, mushroom, pickle, and cucumber rolls, and allowed ourselves two pieces of smoked salmon sushi Dessert: Italian ice Beverage: beer
Hot steel-cut oatmeal with flax seed, raisins, and maple syrup Beverage: water	Hot vegetable bullion with pasta and Parmesan cheese Beverage: grape juice with seltzer	Fresh salad of radicchio, pea shoots, tomatoes, and shallots, served with homemade no-oil dressing Beverage: glass of red wine
Hot ten-grain cereal with flax seed and fresh sliced strawberries Beverage: orange juice	Vegetable pizza Beverage: grape juice with seltzer	Pasta primavera of penne with grilled vegetables, sprinkled with Parmesan cheese Beverage: glass of red wine
Hot steel-cut oatmeal with flax seed, raisins, and maple syrup Beverage: Water	Leftover pasta primavera of penne with grilled vegetables, sprinkled with Parmesan cheese Beverage: grape juice with seltzer	Grilled eggplant rolls, mushroom blinis, and dark bread Dessert: Honey nut cake Beverage: dry martini
Fresh sliced pear	Allowed ourselves pasta with chopped	Vegetable soup puree mixed with black beans

Hot ten-grain cereal with flax seed, raisins, and maple syrup Beverage: orange juice	clams sprinkled with grated Parmesan cheese Beverage: Italian vermouth	Grilled white mushrooms and onions, sautéed spinach, and cous cous Beverage: glass of red wine
Hot steel-cut oatmeal with flax, maple syrup, almond milk, and fresh strawberries Beverage: water	Vegetable soup puree mixed with black eye beans, served with shredded beats and tahini with whole grain toast Beverage: grape juice with seltzer	Fresh garden salad with no-oil dressing Grilled white mushrooms and onions, sautéed spinach, and cous cous Beverage: glass of red wine
Hot ten-grain cereal with flax seed, maple syrup, fresh blueberries, and almond milk Beverage: orange Juice	Veggie burger with lettuce, tomatoes, and olives on nine-grain oat bread Beverage: V-8 Fusion	Pasta with white beans seasoned with homemade pesto sauce of fresh basil, pignoli nuts, minced garlic, and apple sauce Beverage: glass of red wine
Fresh sliced pear Hot ten-grain cereal with flax seed, cinnamon, maple syrup, and almond milk Beverage: orange juice	Angel hair pasta with black olives, sprinkled with grated Parmesan cheese Beverage: grape juice with seltzer	Cooked vegetable salad of beets, carrots, young potatoes, white beans, black beans, corn, and pickled cucumbers, sprinkled with black pepper and Trader Joe's Everyday Seasoning of mustard seed, black peppercorn, coriander, onion, garlic, paprika, and chili Peppers stuffed with rice, sautéed onions, carrots, crushed tomatoes,

		spices, and Trader Joe's beef-less beef made of textured wheat and soy protein Beverage: glass of red wine
Fresh strawberries Beverage: orange juice	Sautéed baby portobello mushrooms with onions and Texas Red spices, served with steamed garlic broccoli and boiled young potatoes Beverage: beer	Fresh mixed greens salad with homemade, nonfat, oil-free dressing, served with whole-wheat toast with tahini (sesame seed) spread Homemade sweet bell peppers stuffed with brown rice, sautéed onions, sautéed carrots, crushed tomatoes, spices, and Trader Joes beef-less beef made of textured wheat and soy protein Beverage: glass of red wine
Fresh strawberries Steel-cut oatmeal with flax seed, cinnamon, maple syrup, and almond milk Beverage: orange juice	Fresh mixed greens salad with homemade, nonfat, oil-free dressing, served with tahini spread on whole-wheat toast Cooked vegetable salad of beets, carrots, young potatos, white beans, black beans, corn, and dill-pickled cucumbers, sprinkled with ground black pepper and	Leftovers of last night's dinner Beverage: grape juice with seltzer

	Trader Joe's Everyday Seasoning of mustard seed, black pepper, coriander, onion, garlic, paprika, and chili Beverage: grape juice with seltzer	
Freshly sliced pear and apple Hot ten-grain cereal with flax seed, raisins, maple syrup, and almond milk Beverage: grape juice with seltzer	Grilled mushrooms and onions, boiled potatoes with tahini, black beans, spicy sliced carrots, and mini Triscuits Beverage: grape juice with seltzer	Sautéed shitaki mushrooms with onions, sautéed spinach with fresh garlic, and mashed sweet potatoes spiced with nutmeg and cinnamon Beverage: glass of red wine
Fresh pear Hot steel-cut oatmeal with flax seed, raisins, maple syrup, and almond milk Beverage: orange juice	Leftovers of last night's dinner Beverage: grape juice with seltzer	Homemade borsch soup of potatoes, parsnip, carrots, onions, tomatoes, cabbage, beets, tomato puree, and black beans, sprinkled with grated Parmesan cheese and served with whole-wheat toast Dessert: piece of dark chocolate Beverage: glass of red wine
Fresh strawberries Hot steel-cut oatmeal with flax seeds, raisins, maple syrup, and almond milk	Leftovers of last night's dinner	Trader Joe's beef-less beef made of textured wheat and soy protein spiced with soyaki sauce, white wine, and curry, served with sautéed zucchini and yellow squash

Beverage: water	Beverage: grape juice with seltzer	Beverage: glass of red wine
Fresh strawberries Hot steel-cut oatmeal with flax seeds, raisins, maple syrup, and almond milk Beverage: water	Allowed ourselves smoked salmon with capers and onions, served with toast points Beverage: glass of white wine	Homemade borsch of potatoes, carrots, onions, tomatoes, cabbage, beets, tomato puree, and black beans, sprinkled with Parmesan cheese and served with whole-wheat toast
Fresh strawberries Hot steel-cut oatmeal with flax, bran, maple syrup, and almond milk Beverage: orange juice	Tahini with Triscuits Beverage: grape juice with seltzer	Olivie salad (potato salad with green peas), a few bites of leftover smoked salmon, Greek salad with feta cheese and roasted potatoes Dessert: Kiev cake Beverage: cranberry juice with seltzer, champagne

So there you have a real picture of our initial meat-free meals. Note that in keeping with our six days a week agreement, we occasionally allowed ourselves seafood, although no more than once a week, typically on Sundays or holidays. And we paired our dinners with our preferred wines and occasional cocktails. The initial goal is not perfect compliance but to move in the direction of healthy meat-free eating without ever feeling deprived. It's not a regime requiring enforcement, but a foodstyle to be gladly embraced.

As interest in the meat-free foodstyle grows, more information is available online, much of it at no cost. People who embrace this foodstyle are usually happy to share their experiences and encourage others to consider trying it.

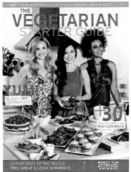 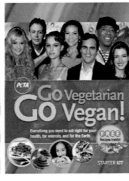

Mercy for Animals (MFA) and People for the Ethical Treatment of Animals (PETA), two outstanding animal welfare organizations with media-savvy advocacy campaigns, make available free starter kits that facilitate an easy entry into adopting a meat-free foodstyle. MFA's is available through http://www.mercy foranimals.org/vegan-starter-kit.aspx. PETA's is available at peta.org/living/food/free-vegetarian-starter-kit.

> Nutrition information in this book is not intended to replace advice from a physician or nutritionist. Discuss any diet changes with your trusted healthcare professional, especially if you have any medical conditions, health challenges, or food allergies.

If you're ready to try making meat-free meals yourself, you'll need to shop for ingredients. Here is what our starter shopping list of some staple items for a meat-free foodstyle looked like. You can re-order items according to your preferences and add foods that you and your family enjoy. It is important to achieve a balance in your food choices to ensure that you are meeting your nutritional requirements while satisfying your palate.

Fruits	Vegetables	Specialty Items
apples	lettuce	mushrooms
bananas	endive	baba ganoush
blueberries	radicchio	guacamole
strawberries	garlic	hummus
raspberries	onions	tahini
peaches	tomatoes	tempeh
pears	cucumbers	natto
kiwis	radishes	miso
tangerines	avocado	apple sauce
oranges	asparagus	agave nectar
lemons	broccoli	maple syrup
limes	brussels sprouts	organic honey
raisins	carrots	molasses
olives	kale	variety of nuts
Bakery	spinach	variety of seeds
pita bread	eggplant	wheat germ
whole-grain bread	zucchini	flax
multi-grain rolls	parsnip	tea
sandwich rolls	squash	coffee
bagels	potatoes	fruitsicles

Beverages	Packaged Foods	Sauces + Spices
almond milk	variety of beans	tomato sauce
soy milk	crackers	pesto sauce
hemp milk	pasta	crushed garlic
grape juice	rice	Dijon mustard
orange juice	quinoa	low-sodium soy sauce
apple cider	couscous	teriyaki sauce
pineapple juice	polenta	soyaki sauce
tomato juice/V-8	hot oatmeal	apple cider vinegar
blueberry juice	cold cereal	red wine vinegar
seltzer water	popcorn	rice vinegar
beer	dark chocolate	salad seasoning
wine	protein shake mix	extra virgin olive oil
Liqueurs	favorite herbs	preferred spices

10
BUON APPETITO

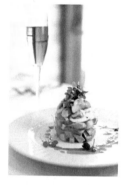

Ease yourself into the transition to a meat-free foodstyle by starting with simple-to-prepare meals, such as rich, colorful soups with lots of different ingredients or vegetable casseroles served with tasty garlic bread. Then try grilled veggie burgers on toasted hamburger buns or veggie meatballs simmered in a spicy Italian sauce on your favorite pasta. Finally, move on to more complex dishes such as grilled portobello mushrooms served with lemon-steamed asparagus and a side of quinoa topped with sautéed onions.

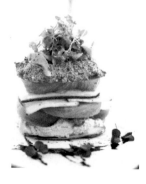

If you need some inspiration, visit some vegetarian or vegan restaurants to see how appealing, delicious, and nutritious meat-free meals can be. The photos on this and the next page are three tasty examples, all gluten-free, courtesy of two of my favorite vegan venues in Manhattan — Candle 79 and Candle Cafe West. The first is Avocado

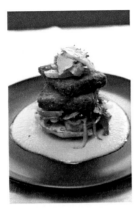 Tomato Tartare made with avocado, tomatoes, cucumber, vegetable and wild mushroom ceviche, and jalapeno dressing. The second is Live Lasagna made with heirloom tomatoes, zucchini, wild mushrooms, cashew cheese, pine nut pesto, and a balsamic black pepper reduction. The third is Cornmeal-Crusted Tempeh made with cornmeal crusted tempeh, sauteed poblano peppers, onions, potatoes, corn sauce, and grilled peach salad.

After you have feasted on some professionally prepared vegetarian and vegan cuisine, you will not be able to think of meat-free meals as boring or tasteless. Quite the contrary: you will be amazed at how robust the flavors are of foods that you may have overlooked your entire life.

A whole new world of experimentation in your own kitchen will open up to you. Most of the meals can be prepared quickly and easily and, without the inclusion of meat, they can be very budget friendly.

You will find the transition easier if you plan your meals and prepare a weekly shopping list. You may also want to cook enough of a meal so it can be served as leftovers the next day. The idea is to make your food prep easy so that a meat-free foodstyle fits in seamlessly with your family's lifestyle.

If your supermarket doesn't carry all of the items you seek, you may have to buy some things at shops specializing in organic foods. More are opening across the country as the meat-free foodstyle catches on, although some neighborhoods still lack food stores with a broad enough inventory of healthier foods. Whether you jump into the meat-free foodstyle quickly or gradually, your confidence will grow as you create your own combinations that please your palate, enhance your health, and save animals' lives.

When dining at restaurants, you may want to read the menu more carefully than usual in order to ensure that you don't accidentally order an appetizer or entree that contains meat or is served with a meat sauce. If in doubt, ask your wait staff. You have a right to know what's in your food. It's been my experience that most wait staff will willingly share that information.

Whether eaten at home or in a restaurant, meals are meant to be enjoyed. Allow yourself to experience the subtle and nuanced flavors that may have previously escaped your appreciation. Embrace the increased mental clarity and energy that you'll soon begin to feel without animal fats polluting your bloodstream. And reflect upon the knowledge that no fellow creature had to give up his or her life so that you could eat. This will reinforce that you made the right decision in adopting a meat-free foodstyle.

11
THE LIVES YOU WILL SAVE

Adopting a meat-free foodstyle is a "switching" of our food choices, not a "sacrificing" of anything required for our human purpose or pleasure. What we gain by making such a switch is in our own self-interest. We enhance our health by eliminating animal flesh, reducing the risk of chronic diseases such as arteriosclerosis, cancer, diabetes, and obesity. In eating more vegetables, legumes, fruits, nuts, and seeds, we improve the nourishment of our bodies, enhance our metabolism, experience greater energy and mental clarity, and, for many people, improve our health measures enough to reduce dependence on some long-term medications. The net effect of these benefits is to improve the quality of our lives and, perhaps, their length. In short, the first life you save by adopting a meat-free foodstyle will be your own.

As societies move in this direction, the supply-and-demand calculus will gradually change, with less land and fewer resources devoted to raising and slaughtering animals and more redirected to growing nutritious plant-based foods. Over time, as industrial agriculture practices change, so too should government polices that impact trade, investment, and foreign aid. Changing food consumption patterns in the developed world holds the potential to allow the developing world the opportunity to grow enough nutritious plant-based food to feed its own malnourished populations. So the second life you save by adopting a meat-free foodstyle could be a fellow human being you will never meet but whose capacity to hunger is no different than your own.

Adopting a meat-free foodstyle will save the lives of innocent animals who suffer unimaginable cruelty that not only denies them a natural full life but also prevents them during their shortened lives from fulfilling the behaviors natural to their species. For most of us who don't live near farm animals, it is hard to comprehend that these rarely seen fellow creatures are not "things" but "beings"—living, breathing, playful, affectionate creatures whose languages we humans don't understand and, consequently, whose protests against our cruelty go unheeded. I invite you to meet some of the animals whose lives you will save by adopting a meat-free foodstyle.

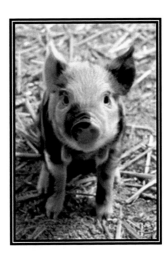

It's common knowledge that pigs are intelligent creatures. But how intelligent? According to Cambridge University Veterinary School Professor Donald Broom, "Pigs have the cognitive ability to be quite sophisticated. Even more so than dogs and certainly [more so than human] three-year-olds." At Penn State University, Professor Stanley Curtis has found that pigs can play joystick-controlled video games and are capable of abstract representation. Suzanne Held of the University of Bristol's Centre of Behavioural Biology says that pigs are "really good at remembering where food is located." Biologist and Johannesburg Zoo Director Lyall Watson writes in *The Whole Hog,* "I know of no other animals [who] are more consistently curious, more willing to explore new experiences, more ready to meet the world with open mouthed enthusiasm."

Pigs use at least twenty different sounds to communicate, from expressing hunger to courting a mate. They have a good sense of direction, which enables them to find their way home. They are affectionate and snuggle. Unlike on factory farms, in their natural surroundings, pigs play, sun bathe, and explore. Pigs rescued to sanctuaries enjoy playing with soccer balls. Piglets recognize and run toward their mothers' voices, and mother pigs sing to their young while nursing.

If we could understand pigs' communications, they would probably ask us to stop killing and roasting them, stop putting them on the barbecue, and stop thinking of their body parts as pork chops, slices of ham, and slabs of bacon. Instead, they would likely encourage us to see them not unlike how we see our dogs. We don't eat them; we play with them.

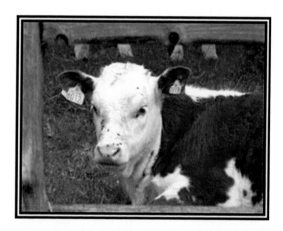

Cows vary widely in personality and intelligence, not unlike humans. Some are curious, adventurous, and bold, while others are shy, timid, and reserved. Cows can hear high and low frequencies better than humans can and can smell odors up to four miles away. According to the Humane Society of the United States, if an individual cow in a herd is shocked by an electric fence, the other cows learn to avoid the fence. Tests conducted by Cambridge University Veterinary School Professor Donald Broom found that cows get excited when they are able to problem solve and overcome obstacles.

Under natural circumstances, cattle live in herds with social hierarchies and form lifelong bonds. As reported by the Montreal-based Global Action Network, researchers have discovered that cows become visibly distressed after being even just briefly separated from a loved one. When permanently separated from their families, cows grieve. The bond formed between a mother and her calf remains long after the calf has grown into adulthood. Farmers well know that mother cows frantically call and search for their calves for days after their calves have been sold off to veal farms.

If a cow spoke in a language that we humans understood, I would imagine that she would tell us that she does not want to be imprisoned on a factory farm, prematurely killed, and have her body cut up and cooked as a steak, a roast, prime rib, or hamburger, or as a brisket to make pastrami and corned beef. She would ask us to stop eating her and let her live her natural life as we wish to live our own.

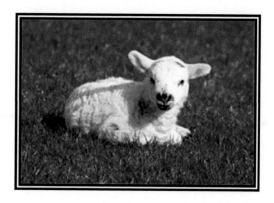

Sheep have a reputation for being among the least intelligent animals, largely due to their timidity and flock instinct, since they have no other means of protection from predators. Researchers have been finding that some of our behavioral assumptions are flawed. Sheep are smart enough to recognize when a sheep in their flock, or a person who regularly cares for them, is absent. They know when an unknown sheep joins their flock.

National Geographic News reported in November 2001 that a team of British scientists had shown that sheep are able to recognize individual faces of fifty sheep and remember them for more than two years. According to Keith Kendrick of the Babraham Institute in England and an author of a report published in the November 2001 issue of the journal *Nature,* "If sheep have such sophisticated facial recognition skills, they must have much greater social requirements than we thought." Tests reveal that 80 percent of the time sheep are able to accurately recognize familiar faces. Reports from Australia indicate that sheep know their way around a maze even when the maze is changed, something that took monkeys far longer to learn in similar tests.

Socially, sheep have a strong bias for their own breed and exhibit distress when mixed with other sheep breeds. Sheep are less aggressive when the flock is well represented by both genders. Anecdotally, BBC News reported in July 2004 that villagers in the Yorkshire Moors of England recounted how hungry sheep taught themselves to roll eight feet across hoof-proof metal cattle grids to raid villagers' gardens. According to one witness, "They lie down on their side or sometimes their back and just roll over and over the grids until they are clear. I've seen them doing it. It is quite clever, but they are a big nuisance to the villagers."

If we could converse with sheep, I imagine they would tell us to stop slitting their throats and roasting them; to stop lusting after leg of lamb, hogget, and mutton; and to just let them happily live their natural lives within their grazing flocks.

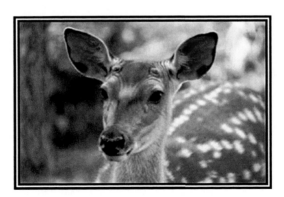

There are many species of deer, including different varieties of deer, moose, elk, caribou, and reindeer. Deer are very cautious animals with well-developed senses of sight, smell, and hearing. The musculature attached to their ears enables them to turn their ears in any direction without moving their heads. Deer can perceive higher sound frequencies than humans. With their eyes positioned on the sides of their head, deer have up to a 310-degree view, though this positioning renders them less able to focus on a single point.

Some deer species are social while others live solitary lives. Male deer—known as bucks, bulls, or stags—tend to be loners, except during the breeding season, known as the rut, when they seek female deer—called does, cows, or hinds. Does often travel together, accompanied by their young. They give birth in summer to one to three fawns at a time after a gestation period of seven months. Their offspring are scentless their first few days to avoid detection by predators and remain with their mothers for up to two years.

When a deer senses danger, he will first try to quietly sneak away. If seriously threatened, he will sometimes make a loud blowing sound and quickly run away with his tail raised like a flag to warn other deer. A whitetail deer can run up to forty miles per hour and swim over ten miles per hour. Not unlike all caring parents, does teach their fawns at an early age to avoid danger and how to hide and be still when threatened. The average life expectancy of an unhunted deer is twenty years.

If we could develop a dialogue with a deer, she would presumably encourage us to appreciate her grace and beauty, but to stop lusting after her relatives as venison steak, burgers, and chops. And she would certainly tell us to stop mounting their heads on our mantles and walls.

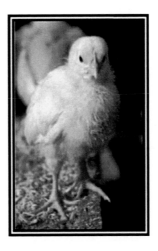

Chickens were domesticated eight thousand years ago. There are about 150 varieties today. Although they are birds, their longest recorded flight is only thirteen seconds, evidence that these birds are incapable of sustained flight. Chickens can, however, walk at speeds of up to nine miles per hour. They are also very social animals and can recognize at least one hundred different faces. Researchers have documented twenty different calls in their vocabulary, including the ability to express different alarms.

Chickens fight to protect family members and mourn when one is lost. When a rooster finds something good to eat, he may call other chickens, particularly his hen, to eat first. He does this by clucking in a high pitch and picking up and dropping the food.

Chickens build private nests to birth their young. A mother hen first scratches a hole in the ground, and then picks up twigs and leaves that she uses to line the rim of the hole. It takes a hen twenty-four hours to lay an egg, which can vary in color from white, to brown, to green, to pink, to blue. The color of a hen's first egg is the color that she will lay for her entire life. Once an egg is laid, it takes twenty-one days for a chick to develop.

The mother hen begins bonding with her chicks before they are born. She turns her egg as often as five times an hour and clucks to her unborn chicks who chirp back to her and to one another. When left undisturbed by humans, chickens can live for five to ten years, and hens from fifteen to twenty years.

If chickens could speak in human languages, they would tell us to stop broiling their breasts, frying their wings, and eating their thighs, that there is no such thing as chicken fingers, and that all they want to do is live.

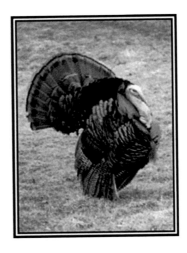

Wild turkeys can fly short distances at speeds up to fifty-five miles per hour and can run at twenty-five miles per hour. Unfortunately, domesticated turkeys are forced to gain up to twice the normal weight of a wild turkey, rendering them unable to fly and denying them this behavior natural to their species.

Even though turkeys have no external ears, they have excellent hearing. Not unlike humans, turkeys also see in color. Turkeys have a wide field of vision of 270 degrees and can see movement one hundred yards away in light, but don't see well at night.

Turkeys are social animals, enjoy the company of other creatures including humans, and like having their feathers stroked, not unlike how dogs like to be scratched. Each spring, male turkeys

spread their tail feathers and make gobbling sounds to attract fe-
males. After mating, a female makes a nest under a bush and lays
her eggs, one each day until she has a complete clutch of eight to
sixteen eggs. After about twenty-eight days, the chicks hatch and
flock with their mother for their first year of life.

Referring to turkeys as "birds of courage," Benjamin Franklin
wanted the turkey to be named as the national bird of the United
States, instead of the bald eagle.

If we could "talk turkey" with turkeys, they would tell us to stop
imprisoning them, stop pumping them with drugs, stop turning
them into obese caricatures of their wild ancestors, and stop putting their corpses on our holiday dinner tables. And they may
also tell us to put an end to the mockery of giving a few turkeys
a presidential pardon while fifty million of their brethren are
killed, sliced up, and eaten during each American Thanksgiving.

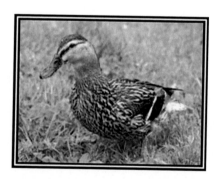

One of the pleasures of childhood is feeding ducks at a pond. Like all animals, ducks are sentient beings with complex behaviors that go unrecognized by most people. Each duck is an individual and is recognized as such by their own kind.

Notwithstanding our perceptions to the contrary, ducks don't mindlessly quack; the pitch and tone of each quack conveys meaning. Moreover, scientists have discovered that ducks have regional accents; for example, city ducks tend to have louder, shouting quacks, while country ducks usually have softer, smoother voices.

Ducks are fastidious creatures and are frequently observed preening themselves to keep clean. Ducks are also fast learners. Chicks can swim within a few hours of being born. If they lose their mother, chicks have been known to travel independently as far as a mile to locate water on their own.

Perhaps most remarkable is how ducks, as well as geese, fly in formation. Multiple families of mothers, fathers, goslings (children), and grandparents form gaggles to fly in a formation. This marvel of teamwork and aerodynamic efficient behavior enables the group to fly up to 70 percent farther than if each bird flew solo. When the lead bird tires, they rotate positions in the formation so another takes the lead, while the birds in back honk to encourage those in front to keep up their speed.

As many of us have experienced in hand-feeding them, ducks can trust humans very quickly. If we could understand their aspirations, they would not include being roasted or baked, and certainly not being force-fed to such grotesque proportions that their organs press on their lungs leaving them unable to breathe normally, so we can fatten their livers to make foie gras. They might say to us, "Watch us fly, see us swim, and play with and feed us. But don't abuse us or eat us."

12
SPREADING THE MEAT-FREE FOODSTYLE

If you think the ideas outlined in this book merit consideration, share them with your family, friends, and coworkers. To help spread the message, consider giving copies of this book as gifts to people in your life to help them understand why you eliminated animal flesh from your diet. This might get them to rethink their own dietary choices and lead them on the path to a healthier life and a relationship of authentic friendship with animals. Should you feel inspired, write a review on amazon.com to draw attention to the information in this book. Get involved in an animal welfare or advocacy organization, visit farm animal sanctuaries, or write to your elected representatives to more aggressively enforce laws against animal cruelty and inspections of factory farms. Each of us individually can play a small but important role in changing hearts and minds. Join me and the other wonderful people who enjoy a meat-free foodstyle in advocating on behalf of our fellow voiceless creatures.

Margaret Mead, the world-renowned cultural anthropologist and posthumous 1979 recipient of the Presidential Medal of Freedom, once said, "Never doubt that a small group of thoughtful, committed people can change the world. Indeed, it is the only thing that ever has."

Thank you for lending your voice to the voiceless.

"Animals are counting on compassionate people like you to give them a voice and be their heroes by learning about the issues they face and taking action. Each of us has the power to save animals from nightmarish suffering—and best of all, it's easier than you might think."

Ingrid Newkirk, President of People for the Ethical Treatment of Animals

"Those who have a voice must speak for those who are voiceless."

Archbishop and Martyr Oscar Romero (1917–1980)

IMAGE CREDITS

ABOUT THE AUTHOR

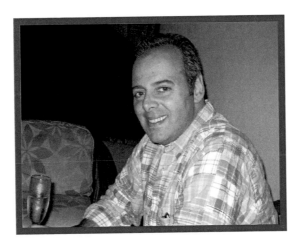

Jerry H. Parisella and his wife, Anna A. Parisella, adopted a meat-free foodstyle in 2011 and quickly experienced more sustained energy, greater mental clarity, easier weight loss, and improved medical test results. They soon came to the profound realization that all animals—in our homes, in the wild, or on factory farms—desire and deserve to live out their full, natural lives. Jerry and Anna are thrilled to share information, experiences and recipes with anyone interested in a meat-free foodstyle.

Jerry is a talent development professional, founder of a live on-line learning company, a former corporate banker, and a United States Air Force veteran. He graduated *summa cum laude* from Gordon College in Massachusetts and earned a Master's Degree from Georgetown University's Walsh School of Foreign Service in Washington, DC. He and his wife currently make their home in New York City with Mishka, their fourth charming and cherished ambassador of the animal kingdom.

StopEatingTheAnimals.org

Made in the USA
San Bernardino, CA
11 June 2018